Exercises In Medical Billing

A Real Life™ Book
Including a Simulated Work Program

ICDC Publishing, Inc.

Los Angeles

Publisher: ICDC Publishing, Inc.
Editor-in-Chief: Sharon E. Brown
Editor: Caitlind L. Alexander
Assistant Editor: Nicole Marie Ghio
Copyeditor: Jennifer Bowen
Copyeditor: Teresa Aguilar
Layout and Design: Anita M. Garcia
Technical Consultant: CarolAnn Jeffries, PA-C, MHS

Third Edition

Copyright © 2005 by ICDC Publishing, Inc.

Printed in the United States of America

ICDC Publishing, Inc.
4123 Lankershim Blvd.
North Hollywood, CA 91602
Phone: (818) 487-1199
Fax: (818) 487-1186
www.ICDCPublishing.com

International Standard Book Number 0-13-169465-0

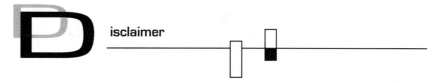

Disclaimer

This manual is a guide for learning and practicing the skills of a medical biller. Decisions should not be based solely on information within this manual. Decisions impacting the practice of medical billing and patient accounting must be based on individual circumstances including legal/ethical considerations, local conditions and payor policies.

The information contained in this manual is based upon experience and research. However, in the complex, rapidly changing medical environment, this information may not always prove correct. Data used are widely variable and can change at any time. Billing personnel should follow current coding regulations outlined by official coding organizations.

The publisher and author do not accept responsibility for any adverse outcome from undetected errors, opinion and analysis contained in this manual that may be inaccurate or incorrect, or from the reader's misunderstanding of an extremely complex topic. All names used in this book are completely fictitious. Any resemblance to persons or companies, current or no longer existing is purely coincidental.

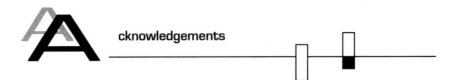

Acknowledgements

Many people have contributed to the development and success of *Exercises In Medical Billing*. We extend our thanks and deep appreciation to the many students and classroom instructors who have provided us with helpful suggestions for this edition of the text.

We would like to express our thanks to the following individuals:

Linda Jepson
Janet Grossfeld, Adelante Career Institute, Van Nuys, CA
Hollis Anglin and Michael Coffin, Dawn Training Institute, New Castle, DE
Michael Williams and Tim McCall, 4-D College, Colton, CA
Anna McCracken and Lynn Russell, American Career College, Los Angeles, CA
Jeff Ward, MediSoft/NDC Health, Mesa, AZ
L'Tanya Knight, Institute of Medical Studies, Irvine, CA

Thanks to the CPA firm of Miller, Kaplan, Arase and Company, LLP:

Mannon Kaplan, C.P.A.
George Nadel Rivin, C.P.A.
Joseph C. Cahn, C.P.A.
Edwin Kanemaru, C.P.A.
Kenneth R. Holmer, C.P.A.
Douglas S. Waite, C.P.A.
Charles Schnaid, C.P.A.
Donald G. Garrett, C.P.A.
Catherine C. Gardner, C.P.A.
Jeffrey L. Goss, C.P.A.

And finally to:

Sean Adams
Sydney Adams
Floree Brown
Nathaniel Brown Sr.

INTRODUCTION

Welcome to the exciting world of medical billing. This book contains a **Real Life™** simulated work program to help you gain the real life experience of a medical biller.

This book is created for use in conjunction with ICDC Publishing's *Guide To Medical Billing*. Some of the exercises in the simulated work portion are based upon concepts learned in the *Guide To Medical Billing* (i.e., procedure and diagnosis coding, privacy issues, etc.). This book should not be considered a complete text for learning medical billing. It is important that trainees not only learn to enter data into a computer billing program, but also to understand the concepts behind what they are entering. It is suggested that a trainee take a complete medical billing course prior to practicing medical billing with this book. The simulated work portion of this text incorporates concepts, which are not taught by simple data entry, for example CPT® and ICD-9 coding, privacy guidelines, patient record keeping, reception area duties, correspondence, and manual completion of claims.

This text is designed to enable you to work through the material at your own pace. The outside margin of this text has been enlarged to allow room for taking notes and jotting down procedure and diagnosis codes.

Section 2 includes training using the MediSoft Patient Accounting software system. MediSoft is one of the most comprehensive and popular computerized medical billing software programs available today. The MediSoft Patient Accounting System not only creates claims for billing insurance carriers, but keeps track of patient accounts and creates most of the forms necessary for running a medical office.

You will need to obtain the MediSoft software program. For further information on MediSoft, or to purchase a copy of their software, please contact MediSoft directly at (800) 333-4747. When using this text, it is important to use MediSoft for **Windows version 5.0** or higher. This text is aimed at using the original version of MediSoft (not the Advanced).

However, this text is **non-version specific.** As such it **may be used with ANY version of MediSoft**. While there have been modifications in the MediSoft program, many of the basic functions have remained the same. In this text we have listed the fields, along with instructions on completing the fields, for each screen. Since your version of MediSoft will probably not include all fields that have ever been used on a screen, simply ignore those that do not apply to your version of the program.

The **Simulated Work Program** contained in Section 3 may be used by students who are using a pegboard or manual system, as well as those using computerized medical billing. Many schools have used the Simulated Work Program with Medical Manager and other computerized medical billing programs. Further information is contained in the Simulated Work Program section. To use an alternate system, simply learn the basics of using the computer system, then skip Section 2 as you go through the text.

On occasion you will be asked to enter data contained in a document (i.e., enter the charges shown on Document 4). All documents are contained in Section 4 of this text. Numerous forms used in the medical office are contained in Sections 5 & 6 in the back of this book and may be copied as needed.

GOOD LUCK as you venture into a challenging, but fulfilling career.

Table of Contents

Understanding the Medical Office and Computers

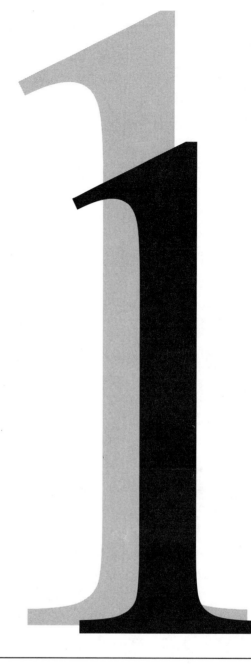

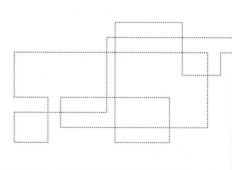

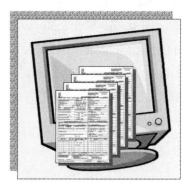

1

Introduction

After completion of this chapter you will be able to:

- Estimate the patient's portion of a bill.
- Set up a patient chart.
- Complete a petty cash count slip.

Let's begin! Today is January 14, 20XX and you have just begun working for Consolidated Health Services (CHS), a large medical care facility. You as a medical biller, keep patient accounts for a number of doctors.

Patients of the offices are often seen by the same doctor each time (their primary care physician [PCP]), but if that PCP is unavailable, or if the patient needs a specialist, they may be referred to another provider within the office group.

After seeing the doctor, patients will often stop by the billing office on their way out to make a payment. At such times the patient's claim information will be given to you, along with a Patient Information Sheet if necessary.

Sue Pervisor is the office manager, and your direct supervisor. While you work in the same office as three other billers, they work on separate accounts. You are responsible for your accounts.

Consolidated Health Services

CHS also owns an inpatient hospital facility. The hospital has an outpatient surgery wing, a lab and x-ray facilities. Attached to one wing of the hospital is a large drug store which sells prescription medications, over-the-counter drugs and some durable medical equipment.

CHS Ambulance Services is a sister company to Consolidated Health Services. While it is a separate entity, it is owned by many of the same partners which own CHS. As such, the billing office also handles bills for the ambulance service.

As a medical biller for CHS, you are responsible for the billing of all doctors in the clinic, the ambulance company, and occasionally for bills from the hospital or drug store (medical equipment charges). It is your responsibility to handle all billing for services rendered and to maintain patient accounts. You will bill the appropriate patients, insurance carriers, Medicare, or other entities responsible for payment; keep track of all patient accounts; make collections calls; and make bank deposits. You may also be asked to watch the front desk for a doctor's receptionist while she is at lunch or on break.

CHS has just begun using the MediSoft Patient Accounting system. Therefore, the system is new to you and all the other medical billers. It is your responsibility to set up the system, and to learn how it works.

Collecting Payments From Patients

Most providers affiliated with CHS choose to collect the patient's portion of the bill after the insurance carrier has made payment. This allows

Drew Blood, M.D.

Reah E. Bright, M.D., (Radiologist)

Noah Pulse, M.D., (Emergency Room)

Kent Cure, M.D., (Emergency Room)

Ben Looney, M.D., (Psychiatrist)

Phil Goode, M.D. (General Practitioner)

Ben Dover, M.D., (Gastroenterologist)

I.D. Liver, M.D., (Obstetrics/Gynecology)

Allotta Payne, M.D., (Obstetrics/Gynecology)

Anne S. Thesia, M.D., (Anesthesiologist)

Yu B. Sickman, M.D., (General Practitioner)

Butch M.N. Hackim, M.D., (Surgeon)

Manny Kutz, M.D., (Assistant Surgeon)

Will Kutteroff, M.D., (Surgeon)

First Floor of Hospital

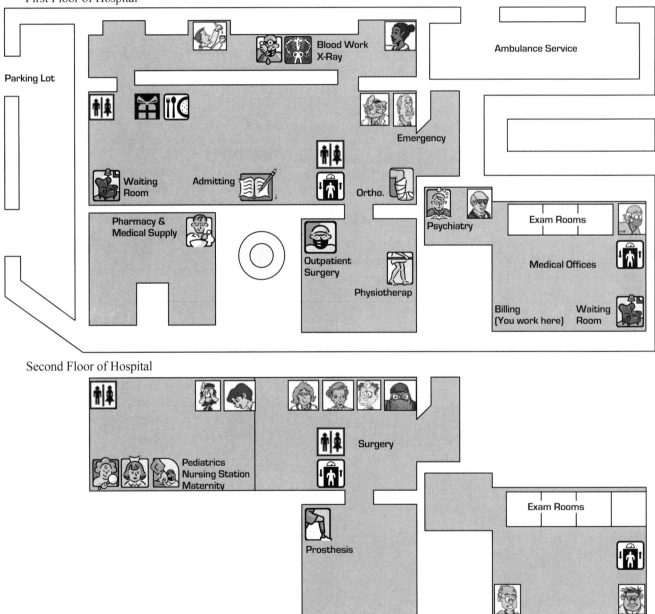

Second Floor of Hospital

The third and fourth floors contain patient rooms and nursing stations.

the billing office to ask for payment from the patient one time only. However, Dr. Ben Dover requests that you estimate the patient's portion of the bill and collect this amount from the patient at the time services are rendered. To do this, you will need to estimate how much the insurance carrier will pay.

First, contact the insurance carrier and determine the deductible amount for the patient, the percent covered by the insurance carrier, and any special payment circumstances. All of this information should be placed on an Insurance Coverage Sheet (see Patient File Forms in Section 6).

The biller should contact the insurance carrier for subsequent visits to determine how much deductible has been previously paid by the patient and how much deductible is left to be paid. Since it is the beginning of the year, many patients will not have met their deductible. To estimate the patient's portion:

1. Subtract the amount of deductible previously met from the yearly deductible amount. This is the amount of deductible remaining to be paid.
2. Subtract the result of step 1 from the total amount of the charges for the visit. This amount will be covered by the insurance at a specified rate (i.e., 80%).
3. Multiply the result of step 2 by the patient's coinsurance amount. For example, if the insurance carrier pays 80% then the patient's coinsurance is 20%.
4. Add the result of step 3 (patient's coinsurance) to the result of step 1 (unpaid deductible). This is the estimated patient responsibility for this bill.

Example: Johnny went to see the doctor for an ear infection. The total charges for services rendered came to $145. You called the insurance carrier and were informed that Johnny's yearly deductible is $100. So far he has met $50.50 of his deductible. The insurance carrier pays 80% and the patient's coinsurance is 20%.

1. $100 (deductible) - $50.50 (deductible paid) = $49.50 (unsatisfied deductible amount).
2. $145 (total charges) - $49.50 (unsatisfied deductible amount) = 95.50 (amount covered by insurance).

3. $95.50 (amount covered by insurance) x 20% (.20; patient coinsurance percentage) = $19.10 (patient's coinsurance amount).
4. $19.10 (patient's coinsurance amount) + $49.50 (unsatisfied deductible amount) = $68.60 (total patient responsibility).

Patients should be informed that additional payments might be necessary if the insurance carrier does not cover the full amount of the bill.

Exercise 1 – 1: Calculate the estimated patient portion for each of the following scenarios.

1. Abby visited the doctor for measles treatment. The total charges came to $230. You called and her insurance carrier informed you that Abby's deductible is $100. So far she has paid $23.25 of her deductible. The insurance carrier pays 80% and the patient's coinsurance amount is 20%.

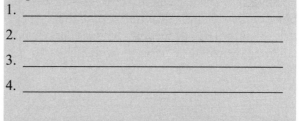

2. Bonnie went to the doctor for the mumps. The total charges came to $195. You called the insurance carrier and were informed that Bonnie's deductible is $150. So far she has met $15 of her deductible. The insurance carrier pays 90%.

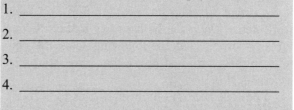

3. Charlie went to the doctor for treatment for whooping cough. The total charges came to $115. You called the insurance carrier and were informed that his deductible is $125. So far he has met $5 of his deductible. The insurance carrier pays 80%.

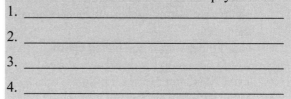

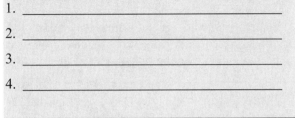

4. Dick went to the doctor for chest pains. The total charges came to $263. You called the insurance carrier and were informed that Dick's deductible is $100. So far he has met $100. The insurance carrier pays 70%.

1. _____

2. _____

3. _____

4. _____

Some computerized billing systems will automatically multiply the amount of the visit by the patient's coinsurance portion. However, they will seldom calculate the amount of the deductible. Many offices prefer not to collect the deductible portion at the time services are rendered since it is possible that another claim for the patient will be processed by the insurance carrier prior to receipt of this claim. The deductible amount previously collected would then need to be refunded to the patient.

Setting Up Your "Office"

Each person going through this text will be responsible for setting up their own office and completing each of the exercises. For this reason it is important to maintain a set of files and other work items which can be used day to day. Setting up your "office" with the following items will help to keep them neat and insure that items are easily accessible.

You will need the following items to properly complete the exercises in this book:

- Two Envelopes (one for Petty Cash/Payments and one for Deposits Made).
- 15 Family/Patient File Folders (see Patient Files section below).
- One "Practice" folder for keeping all daily charts and forms which are generated for the practice.
- One Folder for all completed claims which would be sent to the insurance carrier.
- 110 CMS-1500 forms for billing.
- Five UB-92 forms for billing.

- One Expanding file folder for keeping all of the above items together.
- Pens and pencils.

Additionally, you will need access to the following:
- CPT®, ICD-9, and HCPCS Coding Books,
- Scissors,
- Two- Hole Punch, and
- Medical Dictionary and/or other reference books.

Place the cash and deposit envelopes in the front of the expanding folder, followed by the practice folder and then the patient charts. As you are introduced to each patient and/or their family, create a family chart and place it in your expanding file folder. All other forms for setting up your office are located in Patient File Forms – Section 6.

Petty Cash and Deposit Envelope

As a medical biller, you are responsible for keeping a petty cash envelope and for reconciling the amount in petty cash and the amount collected from patients. At the end of each day you will prepare a deposit slip with all payments received during that day. You should recount the petty cash to insure that the same amount remains at the end of the day as there was at the beginning. Also be sure that the money in petty cash is sufficient for making change for customers.

It is suggested that you keep all petty cash and payments received in a single envelope. When a patient makes a payment, place the check or cash into the envelope. If change is needed, remove the proper change from the envelope. A second envelope should be used for deposits. Clearly label the envelopes **CASH ENVELOPE** and **DEPOSITS MADE**.

Section Five contains simulated petty cash for the cash drawer and forms used for petty cash. Cut out each of the bills and coins and place them in your Cash Envelope. Using a copy of the Petty Cash Count slip, determine the amount of money in your petty cash drawer. Your count should always include the paper currency, all coins and petty cash receipts. This slip should be used each time you reconcile petty cash. During the Simulated Work Portion (Section 3), use a.m. to designate the first counting of petty cash at the beginning of the day and p.m. to designate the count at the end of the day.

How much money is in your petty cash envelope?

Additionally, supervisors such as Sue Pervisor may take up to $20 from petty cash to cover small items needed for the office. Each should sign a petty cash receipt (see File Forms – Section 6) showing the date the money was taken, the amount, and what the money was used for. After purchases are made the receipt and any change left over should be returned to the petty cash drawer. Be sure that the amount of the receipt and the change total the amount that was originally given.

Patient Files

The patient files are also kept in your office. CHS keeps family files for their patients, instead of individual files. Each family file consists of a three or four page file folder with pronged paper fasteners at the top for holding information **(see Figure 1 – 1)**. Each file should contain information in the following order:

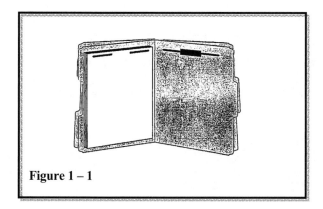

Figure 1 – 1

Fastener 1
1. Patient Information Sheet. (The bottom section of the patient information sheet includes an Authorization to Release Information and an Assignment of Benefits).
2. Insurance Coverage Sheet (This form will be completed and inserted during the Simulated Work Program)

3. Any other forms or information which pertains to the entire family.

Fastener 2
1. Billing information (CMS-1500 claims and patient statements) in chronological order (most recent date first) for the insured. These will be completed during the exercises and simulated work program in this text.

Fasteners 3, 4, and 5
1. Billing information, CMS-1500 claims and patient statements in chronological order (most recent first) for dependents. Each dependent should have their own separate fastener.
2. If there are more than three dependents in the family, insert a divider or folder with fasteners to accommodate the additional family members.

Last Fastener
1. For training purposes, this page will be used to attach all items which are given to the patient or insured. These items can include change for a cash payment, a receipt, or statements, which were sent to the patient.

Patient files should be kept available at all times.

Training tip: For class purposes, you may want to create patient files by placing one manila folder inside another and securing them together at the fold. Then attach a two pronged paper fastener at the top of each page to hold the papers in place. Keep all of your files in an expanding file folder.

Summary

As a medical biller at Consolidated Health Services you have numerous responsibilities. Some of those responsibilities include setting up and maintaining patient billing information, estimating the patient portion of charges, and reconciling petty cash. With practice you will become proficient at these skills and acquire many more making you a valuable member of CHS.

Questions for Review

Directions: Answer the following questions without looking back into the material just covered. Write your answers in the space provided.

1. What is the purpose of a petty cash receipt?

    _____

    _____

2. Name two uses for petty cash.

    1._____

    2. _____

3. List the three items on the petty cash count slip.

    1.   _____

    2.   _____

    3.   _____

4. List the four steps for estimating the patient's portion of a bill.

    1.   _____

    2.   _____

    3.   _____

    4.   _____

5. What items are placed on side three of the family chart? _____

    _____

If you were unable to answer any of the questions, refer back to that section, and then fill in the answers.

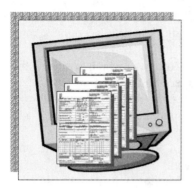

2

Computers –
A Quick Review

After completion of this chapter you will be able to:

- List the three main components of a computer system.
- Describe the keyboard and demonstrate its use.
- Define commonly used computer terms.

In today's world, computers are a common part of life. They are used in nearly every business and in many home environments. In the medical community, computers are used extensively for billing patients, handling patient accounting, and handling the provider's accounts and correspondence.

Computer Terminology

With the development of computers, a whole new set of terms had to be created to define items relating to the application and use of these machines. While "computerese" is a complete language that could take years to understand, the person who uses computers will need to be familiar with a number of terms. The most common of terms include the following.

Back Up – A back up copy is a duplicate file or set of information contained in a different area of the computer or on magnetic tape or disk. This allows you to recreate information if something should happen to your main file.

Batch – A group of documents, papers or forms which are related in some way, often by date or batch number. Unrelated papers or claims may be put together in a batch and given a specific number.

Bit – Binary digit, the smallest possible unit of memory storage. Eight bits is equal to one byte.

Bug – A computer program error. Bugs can cause a program to work improperly, or not at all.

Byte – A measurement for the storage capacity of computers. A byte is equal to eight bits, or roughly the amount of bits needed to make one character or letter.

Central Processing Unit (CPU) – The brains of a computer. It controls the internal memory and directs the processing and flow of information.

Command Key – A key or combination of keys, which activates a command in a computer program.

Cursor – A small light, bar or flashing line on the computer screen, which indicates the position of the next data entry.

Data Base – A collection of electronically stored data.

Debug – To remove errors from a computer or a software program.

Disk – A device for storing information. There are two main types of disks: hard and floppy.

> **Disk, Hard** – A disk made of hard material that can be stored inside the computer housing or outside, attached securely by cables and wires.
>
> **Disk, Floppy** – A plastic diskette which holds data information and is easily transportable. Floppy disks are often 3.5 inches square. Compact discs (CDs), are replacing 3.5 inch disks as they are easier to transport, more durable, and can hold more information.

Documentation – An instruction book detailing how to use a computer program.

DOS – Disk Operating System. A set of programmed instructions which commands the computer's operation.

Down Time – The time during which a computer is not operating properly.

Footer – A notation which appears at the bottom of a page or computer screen.

Format – The way the data is organized or how it appears. Format can include whether items are presented in upper or lower case, numbered or lettered, left, center or right aligned, width of margins, or many other factors.

Hard Copy – A print-out of information from the computer.

Hardware – The pieces or components of a computer system. These can include the monitor, keyboard, hard disk, computer housing, or modem.

Header – A notation which appears at the top of a page or computer screen.

Input – To enter information into a computer.

Interface – The linking of two or more computer systems (i.e., computer to computer, or computer to printer).

K (kilobyte) – A unit of memory storage measurement. A K is equal to 1,000 bytes. For example, a computer may have 640 K of memory.

Memory – The computers ability to store data.

Menu – A list of items or computer functions displayed on a computer screen from which the operator can choose.

Modem – A device which converts outgoing digital data into sound waves so it can be transmitted across telephone lines, and which can reconvert incoming sound waves into digital data. Most computers have a built in "internal" modem.

Mouse – A hand-held device used to control the video display of a computer.

Network – An interconnection of computers.

On-line System – 1) A system where data is input directly into the computer and output data is sent directly from the computer to where it is used (i.e., printer, modem). 2) A system which works without human intervention between the recording and the processing of material.

Optical Character Recognition (OCR) – A device which can read typed characters and convert them to computer data.

Program – Another word for software; a set of instructions which can be loaded into the computer.

It commands the computer on how to work to achieve the purposes of the program (i.e., MediSoft is a program for medical patient accounting and billing).

Prompt – A symbol (often >) which indicates the computer is ready to receive information.

RAM (Random Access Memory) – A data storage system in which data may be stored randomly, and retrieved by specifying its location.

Retrieve – The act of locating a stored file and bringing it up on screen.

ROM (Read-Only Memory) – A data storage system in which information can be read, but not changed. This usually includes permanent programs.

Scrolling – The ability to move from one side of the screen to another, top to bottom, or page by page through a document.

Soft Copy – The information displayed on a computer screen. The printing of this data onto paper is called a hard copy.

Software – Another word for computer program.

Sort – The process by which a computer arranges data in a specified order.

Spooling – A device whereby the output from a computer is placed in storage queues to await transmission to a device which moves slower than the computer output (i.e., the storage of data to a file until it can be read by a printer with a more limited memory capacity).

Terminal – A device or system which can receive information from and send information to a computer system.

Time-sharing – The use of a computer device for more than one purpose at one time (i.e., working on one document while another is being sent to the printer) or the use of a system by more than one user at one time.

Voice Activation – The ability of a computer device to recognize and respond to verbal commands.

The Computer

There are three main components to a computer, the central processing unit, the monitor, and the keyboard. The central processing unit is enclosed in a box which houses the memory and functional components of the computer. The monitor is the screen connected to the computer. This screen allows you to see the program and the data you are working with. The keyboard is the primary means of communicating with the computer. The input commands and data are typed through the keyboard.

Since the keyboard is the main component used to enter data, we will describe it in more detail. There are five main parts of a keyboard: the angle adjustment, the typewriter keypad, the numeric keypad, the shortcut keys, and the function keys.

The keyboard angle adjustment consists of two small legs which are located under the back of the keyboard. Pushing these up or down allows you to adjust the keyboard to two different positions.

The typewriter keypad looks and works like a standard typewriter keyboard. There are alphabetic, numeric and symbol keys, as well as those for spacing and capitalizing letters.

The numeric keypad is usually located on the right-hand side of the keyboard, and performs a dual function. With the Num Lock key engaged it is used for the rapid entry of numbers. Without engaging Num Lock the keypad can be used the same as the shortcut keys.

Between the typewriter keypad and the numeric keypad are the shortcut keys. These keys allow you to move more quickly through a document. These can include the following keys:

- **Home:** Moves you to the beginning of the line the curser is on.
- **End:** Moves you to the end of the line the curser is on.
- **Page Up:** Moves you up one page in the current document.
- **Page down:** Move you down one page in the current document.
- **Delete:** Deletes characters typed to the right of where the cursor is.
- **Insert:** New characters typed in will replace the existing characters shown on the screen.
- **Arrow Keys:** These keys allow you to move the curser one space to the right, left, up, or down in the document.

Function keys allow complex program commands to be performed with a single keystroke. The 12 function keys are located along the top or on the left side of the keyboard. Different software programs use the function keys for different purposes. To properly use them, consult the user manual for the specific program you are working with.

Using the Computer

Different computer systems use different keys to produce the same results. Often if you have mastered one computer system, you will find a related computer system to be fairly easy to learn.

Choosing **main menu options** is the same as choosing a main heading on a restaurant menu. Do you want a main dish today or a salad? Do you want to edit information, or print reports? To choose a main menu option, click on the menu choice at the top of the screen.

Once you have chosen a main menu option, a **submenu option** menu will appear on the screen. Submenu options give you different choices which have been grouped under the main heading. For example, if you chose a salad from the main menu, which type of salad do you prefer, Chinese chicken or chef's salad? If you have chosen to print reports, do you want to print an insurance aging report or a patient ledger?

Disk drives are where the data on your computer is stored. Most personal computers have a **hard drive** installed within the computer. This is most commonly called the C drive. The A and D drives are located on the front of the computer (though some computers only have an A drive installed). The A and D disk drives have a slot through which you can slide a **floppy disk** or **CD.**

A floppy disk is a circular piece of magnetic film which is enclosed in a square plastic holder. When you store information to your disk (i.e., to the A or B drive), you are actually instructing the computer to record the information in your document onto the magnetic film. This is very similar to recording a voice on a cassette tape.

The magnetic field contained in these disks is very sensitive and should be handled carefully. The following rules should be observed when dealing with data diskettes:

1. Never touch the magnetic media housed inside the plastic cover or on the back of the CD.
2. Store all disks or CDs inside a plastic or paper cover to protect them. Insert and remove the disk or CD carefully from the cover to prevent scratching the magnetic media.
3. Keep diskettes stored at temperatures between 50 degrees and 125 degrees

Fahrenheit. Never leave a data disk exposed to sunlight.

4. Keep all magnets away from your data disks. Information is stored on a magnetic media which can be erased when it comes in contact with a magnet. This includes the magnet contained in office supplies such as paper clip holders.

5. Before touching a data disk, discharge any static electricity you may have picked up by touching a piece of metal or an anti-static mat. Static electricity will also demagnetize items and therefore erase the data contained on a disk.

6. To prevent any changes to stored information, cover the "write protect" notch on the side of the disk. On a 3.5 inch disk, this notch can be closed by sliding a small plastic square up to cover the hole.

7. Do not write on a disk label with a ball point pen or pencil, use a felt tip marker.

The pressure applied when writing with pen or pencil may cause impressions on the magnetic media damaging the content.

When information is stored on a disk, the disk can be taken from one computer to another and the data used wherever you would like.

Summary

Computers have infiltrated all aspects of business life, including the medical office. Using the computer saves time, produces neater and cleaner reports, reduces errors, and allows for electronic submission of data to the insurance carrier.

Learning to use a computer program quickly and accurately, and learning the proper means of storing information is important to become a proficient medical biller.

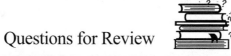

Questions for Review

Directions: Answer the following questions without looking back into the material just covered. Write your answers in the space provided.

1. List the three main components of a computer system and define their use.

    1. _____
    2. _____
    3. _____

2. List the five main parts of the keyboard and define their use.

    1. _____
    2. _____
    3. _____
    4. _____
    5. _____

3. What does it mean to "back up" your data? _____

    _____

    _____

4. The cursor is _____

    _____

    _____

5. Define the following terms:

    RAM _____

    ROM _____

    Menu _____

    Mouse_____

If you were unable to answer any of the questions, refer back to that section, and then fill in the answers.

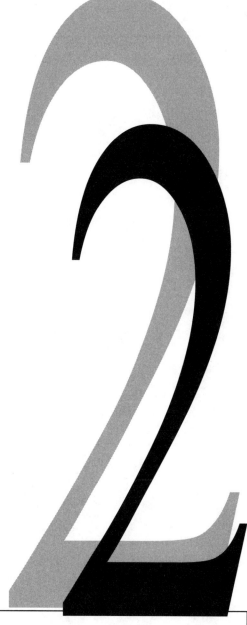

SECTION

Understanding the Computer Program

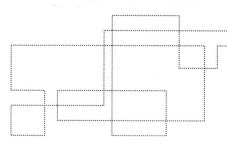

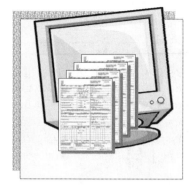

3

Using MediSoft

After completion of this chapter you will be able to:

- Enter and exit the MediSoft program.
- Access menu bar options and select a menu option.
- Access submenu options under the menu bar.
- Operate the function keys.

MediSoft is one of the most comprehensive and popular computerized medical billing software programs available today. The MediSoft Patient Accounting System not only creates claims for billing insurance carriers, but keeps track of patient accounts and creates many of the forms necessary for the efficient running of a medical office.

Due to the constant revising of MediSoft, you may not have the most recent version. In this text we have given you the information about the 2004 version of MediSoft, but we have also included descriptions of menus, fields, and options that are found in earlier versions. The differences among versions are often small and involve renaming a field or repositioning a field within a screen. As you go through your software with this text, keep in mind that something that has been renamed in the new version will most likely have the same function as in the old version.

This text is based on the concept that you learn by doing. Therefore, as you read about each function and field in the MediSoft system, you will also be asked to enter data into these fields. It is important that you take your time and enter the data correctly as it will be used in the simulated work program. If data has been incorrectly entered here, it may adversely affect reports, charges, or other entries which are completed during the simulated work program.

It takes practice to use a computer program quickly and effectively. Do not rush through the exercises. While you will have the opportunity to enter data in each of the screens, these exercises are meant to familiarize you with the screens. Do not worry if you do not feel totally comfortable with the screen. You will gain additional practice using each of the screens during the simulated work program.

Entering MediSoft

To begin using MediSoft, you must first access the system. You should have a MediSoft icon (little picture) on your screen with the word MediSoft underneath. Using your mouse, click on the MediSoft icon. (To "click on" an icon, move the mouse so that the arrow is on the icon and click the left button on the mouse rapidly twice.) The system will then display the MediSoft main screen.

The main screen consists of Menu Bars arranged across the top of the screen. A second level shows icons for accessing specific tools in the MediSoft program.

In previous versions of MediSoft, the main screen displayed five icons:

Uninstall MediSoft Patient Accounting. This key deleted the program from your computer. You **DO NOT** want to hit this button.

MediSoft Patient Accounting. This icon accessed the MediSoft program. It was the icon used most often.

Read Me. This icon lists computer hardware requirements and is used by those setting up the program to insure they can install it properly.

File Maintenance. This option was for recalculating patient balances, purging (or deleting) old data, rebuilding your files, or packing data (making it fit into less disk space).

The **Office Hours** program was previously accessed using this icon. The Office Hours Program is now a separate icon on most desktop screens. This program allows you to set up appointments and keep a calendar for the providers and others in the office. This will be described in more detail in Chapters 10 – 11.

Menu Bar

Before entering data, let's become familiar with the Menu Bar and its options. MediSoft is set up using both a Menu Bar to bring up a menu of options and a Tool Bar for quick access into some of the MediSoft operations. There are nine menu operations in the 2004 version. They are:

1. File
2. Edit
3. Activities
4. Lists
5. Reports
6. Tools
7. Window
8. Help
9. Services

In order to access an item in the Menu Bar, you have two options:
1. Use your mouse to move the arrow to the menu choice and click the button once; or
2. Hold down the Alt key and press the letter which is underlined for each of the menu options.

Accessing each of the choices in the Menu Bar allows you to see the submenu items which can be chosen in that menu option. A list of choices will pop up on the screen from which you may choose. In order to enter a menu choice, access the option by using either of the two methods mentioned above.

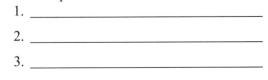

Exercise 3 – 1: Start your computer and enter the MediSoft program. Click on each of the following menu choices as they are discussed, and answer the questions asked. Remember that different versions will vary. Some menus may have fewer choices than there are lines to be filled depending on your version of MediSoft.

The **File Menu** allows the user to enter data regarding the office, backup and restore data, program options, and maintain files. The File Menu's submenu choices are:
1. Open Practice
2. New Practice
3. Backup Data
4. View Backup Disks
5. Restore Data
6. Set Program Date
7. Practice Information
8. Program Options
9. Security Setup
10. File Maintenance
11. Exit

The **Edit Menu** is for editing items. These are usually text items.

List the submenu choices for the Edit Menu in the spaces below.

1. _____
2. _____
3. _____
4. _____

The **Activities Menu** provides an opportunity to enter transactions (billings and payment receipts) and appointments. These are the screens that will be used most often in daily practice.

List the submenu choices in the Activities Menu in the spaces below.

1. _____
2. _____
3. _____

The **Lists Menu** gives you access to lists of those people and entities your practice does business with. These lists usually include names, addresses, and phone numbers, as well as other pertinent data.   List the submenu choices in the Lists Menu in the spaces below.

1. _____

2. _____

3. _____

4. _____

5. _____

6. _____

7. _____

8. _____

9. _____

10. _____

11. _____

The **Reports Menu** allows you to print reports on both the patient and the office. These reports help you keep track of how the practice is doing.

List below the submenu choices in the Reports Menu, including the options given through side arrows.

1. _____

   A. _____

   B. _____

   C. _____

2. _____

   A. _____

3. _____

   A. _____

   B. _____

   C. _____

   D. _____

   E. _____

   F. _____

   G. _____

4. _____

5. _____

6. _____

7. _____

8. _____

9. _____

The **Tools Menu** gives you access to additional tools which might be helpful in making the practice run smoothly.

List below the submenu choices for the Tools Menu.

1. _____

2. _____

3. _____

4. _____

5. _____

6. _____

7. _____

The **Window Menu** allows you to close all open windows.

List below the submenu choices in the Window Menu.

1. _____

2. _____

3. _____

4. _____

5. _____

The **Help Menu** allows you to get more information which you may find helpful in working with MediSoft.

List below the submenu choices in the Help Menu, including the options given through side arrows.

1. _____

2. _____

3. _____

4. _____

5. _____

A. _____

B. _____

C. _____

D. _____

E. _____

6. _____

7. _____

8. _____

The **Services Menu** offers a link to an online resource that allows a practice to write prescriptions over the Internet. These prescriptions can be transmitted to nearby pharmacies, allowing patients to pick up their prescriptions quickly.

List below the submenu choice in the Services Menu.

1. _____

Tool Bar

The Tool Bar is used to quickly access functions. For example, the first icon in the tool bar is for Transaction Entry. If you wish to enter transactions you may click on this icon, or you can click on the Activities Menu, and then choose Enter Transactions.

As you move the mouse arrow to each of the icons, their function will be highlighted both at the site of the icon, and at the bottom of the screen.

For example, the second icon is Claim Management. The wording near the icon says Claim Management. The description at the bottom of the page says "Use this window to print and send insurance claims."

Use your mouse to move the arrow to each of the icons on the Tool Bar. Allow the mouse arrow to rest on the icon a moment. List below the wording that appears near the icon and at the bottom of the screen. (If no wording appears near your icon, this option may be turned off. To turn it on, click on the Help Menu, then choose the Show Hints submenu option. This is an on/off key. A check mark by the option means the hints will be shown. No check means the hints will not show.)

ICON   Identify the ICON and the message that appears at the bottom of the screen

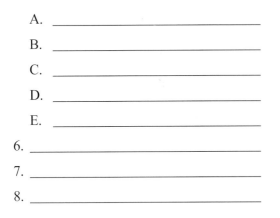

_____

_____

_____

_____

_____

_____

_____

_____

_____

_____

_____

_____

_____

_____

_____

_____

_____

_____

_____

_____

_____

_____

Sidebar Options

If the option to show Sidebar has been checked, your screen may show four subject tabs vertically arranged on the left side of the screen. These are:

1. **Accounting**
2. **Patient Management**
3. **Office Management**
4. **Daily Reports**

Clicking on these tabs opens a menu of more specific options under each heading. These submenu options are the same as those accessed through the main menu bar. Click on each option and list the submenu options below.

The **Accounting sidebar** allows you to perform accounting functions. List below the submenu options found on the Accounting side bar.

1. _____

2. _____

The **Patient Management sidebar** allows you to access options that deal with managing the practice's patients. List below the submenu options found on the Patient Management side bar.

1. _____

2. _____

3. _____

4. _____

The **Office Management sidebar** allows you to access functions, which help the office to run smoothly. List below the submenu options in the Office Management side bar.

1. _____

2. _____

3. _____

4. _____

5. _____

6. _____

7. _____

The **Daily Reports sidebar** allows you to print reports that are used on a daily basis. List below the submenu options in the Daily Reports side bar.

1. _____

2. _____

3. _____

General Functions and Keys

The following functions and keys work on many screens throughout the menus in the MediSoft Patient Accounting system. In MediSoft the available function keys are shown in the command line at the bottom of the screen. They can be used in virtually any screen.

F1 – Help. Pressing this key will give you more information regarding the field that is currently highlighted by the cursor. You may also access this option by clicking on the Help tool bar icon or the Help Menu Option.

F3 – Save. The information entered into each field is not saved until the **F3** key is pressed. This saves the information onto the hard drive and allows it to be retrieved at a later date. If you do not press **F3** at the end of a screen or click on the save button, your data when be lost when you leave that screen.

F6 – Search. The search option is available to search name and description fields. It is not available for use in most numbered fields. The search function works for any string of letters that matches those that are entered. Therefore, if you enter the letters "Jack" in the patient chart/name field, the computer will bring up everything with this string of letters in the beginning of the last name, including Thomas Jackman and Bob Jackson. If you enter a single letter, the computer locates all records that contain that letter in the beginning of a word. Thus, entering "A" in the procedures screen will bring up adjustment, but not cash.

You may also access the search field by clicking on the magnifying glass that is found to the right of many fields.

Pressing **F2** while in the search mode will allow you to search a different index option. For example, in the Procedure Code Information screen, pressing **F2** will search the code number rather than the description of the procedure. Once you have entered the search screen, the bottom of your screen will tell you if the **F2** option is available for this screen and which field will be searched if you press the **F2** key.

F7 – Ledger. Pressing F7 opens the Quick Ledger window. This window allows you to look at the account of the patient you are currently working on.

F8 – New. This key allows you to enter new information into an appropriate screen. A few fields allow you to switch from one screen to another quickly to add necessary information. For example, if you are working on the Transaction Entry screen and attempt to enter a diagnosis that has not been previously entered into the Diagnosis Code data base, pressing **F8** will allow you to quickly access the Diagnosis Code Entry screen. After entering the information on the diagnosis code, pressing **F3** (save) will take you back to the Transaction Entry screen. The information you have just entered into the Diagnosis Code Entry screen will appear in the diagnosis field on the Transaction Entry screen.

F9 – Edit. This key will allow you to edit or change data which has already been saved.

F11 – Quick Balance. This key will allow you to see balance information for the chosen guarantor. Often the guarantor is the insured. Using this window will allow you to see all balances for the insured and their dependents.

F12 – Office Messenger. This key opens the NDC MediSoft Office Messenger program. This allows you to send a quick message to someone else using the program.

The **F1, F6,** and **F8** keys are context sensitive. This means that choosing them will only access files which are related to the current position of the cursor. Therefore, if your cursor is in the Diagnosis Code position, the Help key will tell you about that field only, the Search key will search only for diagnosis codes, etc.

Esc – Exits you from the screen or field you are in and takes you back to the previous menu. Be sure to save prior to pressing **Esc** if you wish to keep your data.

Enter – Enters the information into the current field you are working on and move the cursor to the next entry field.

Space – Hitting the space bar will check or uncheck a box when your cursor is in the box.

Arrow Keys – The up and down arrow keys (↑↓) will move the cursor up or down to the previous or the next field on the screen.

The left and right arrow keys (→ ←) will move the cursor to the right and left within the field you are currently in.

End – The End key will move the cursor to the end of the field you are currently working in.

Home – The Home key will move you to the beginning of the field you are currently working in.

Tab – The Tab key will move the cursor around the screen. This is the key which should be used when you have finished entering data in one field and wish to move on to the next field. If you press Enter after completing a field, in many of the screens MediSoft will assume you have completed the entry and wish to exit that screen.

There are other function keys which only work in a specific menu. For example, the F2 key will open the MultiLink window if you are in the Transaction Entry screen. In the List Windows screen the same F2 key will change the value in the field.

Since the function of these keys is specific to a certain field, they will not be discussed here.

The MediSoft Icon or – Box

The MediSoft Icon in the upper-left-hand corner of the screen has additional menu options. Clicking on this icon will list a menu of these options. In previous versions, a – Box occupied the upper-left-hand corner of the screen. The function remains the same.

Minimize and maximize allow you to change the size of the screen you are looking at. Minimize will make it very small. Maximize will enlarge it to fill the entire screen.

Close will end this application and return you to the previous screen or a blank screen. This is the way to exit an application. While hitting **F3** (save) will automatically exit you from some applications, it should not be used if you have not entered any data into the application. Otherwise you will be saving blank screens, thus using memory storage space.

Summary

The MediSoft Patient Accounting system has a wide variety of menus and screens which provide most functions needed for handling patient accounting. Learning the various operations menus and the items contained within those menus is essential to being able to run the MediSoft program efficiently and effectively.

Some keys function the same throughout all MediSoft menus and fields. Learning these keys and how they function will greatly aid in improving data entry time and ease in operating the computer.

Questions for Review

Directions: Answer the following questions without looking back into the material just covered. Write your answers in the space provided.

1. In which menu sidebar option will you find the Enter Transactions submenu choice? _____

_____

2. What is the name of the menu sidebar option to access the screen for entering patient data into the computer?

_____

3. Which key is used to get more information or "help" on how to fill out a particular field? _____

_____

4. Which key is used to save your data? _____

5. What are the three ways of initiating a search?

    1. _____

    2. _____

    3. _____

6. In which menu bar option will you find the Patient Ledger submenu choice? _____

7. In which menu bar option will you find the Insurance Carriers List submenu choice? _____

8. In which menu sidebar option will you find the Appointment Book submenu choice? _____

9. In which menu bar option will you find the Backup Data submenu choice? _____

10. What function does the **F8** key perform? _____

If you were unable to answer any of the questions, refer back to that section, and then fill in the answers.

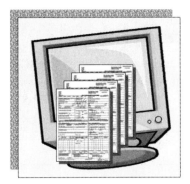

4

File Menu Options

After completion of this chapter you will be able to:

- Set up a practice, set program date, and enter new patient information.
- Restore data, purge unnecessary data, and rebuild your data files.

Now let's actually begin entering data into the system. We will go through each of the menu options one by one. In each you will be asked to enter or change data. Follow the directions exactly and complete each step before moving on to the next. If you skip items, your data could be adversely affected.

The **File Menu** option allows you to enter information pertaining to the practice, change the date, and choose default data. It also allows you to backup and restore data, and contains the File Maintenance option.

Set Program Date

This text contains a simulated work program which will take you through many of the duties a medical biller encounters in a given day. However, in order to make all data match properly, the entry dates for the data will need to be matched.

MediSoft is a date sensitive program and it is important when completing the exercises in this book that you use the date that is given to you. Many operations function using the date entered,

such as the printing of day sheets and other reports. Throughout this text you will be given the date to use.

The Simulated Work Program starts at the beginning of the year so that you can see how deductibles and other items on a patient chart are accumulated. Thus, all initial data which is entered should use the date January 1 of the current year.

Every time you enter the MediSoft program you must be sure you are working on the correct date. Go through each of the following steps each time you begin working on the computer. As you enter the Simulated Work Program part of the course, you will encounter five different days. Be sure to reset the date as you begin each new day which is given in the program. If you do not, your data will not be recorded accurately and your reports will not print properly.

Exercise 4 – 1: Reset the date to January 1, 20XX by doing the following steps:
1. Click on the **File** Menu option.
2. Choose **Set Program Date** by either clicking on it, or by striking **D** (the underlined letter).
3. Click on the (right/left arrows) next to the current month to move backward or forward through the months until you reach January, or click on the month shown and choose a month.
4. If the year is not correct, click on the year shown, and choose 20XX (with XX being replaced by the current year).
5. A January 20XX calendar will appear. Click on the **1** within the date boxes to indicate that this is January 1st.

This will change the date for this use of the program. However, each time you exit the program then go back in, you will need to reset the date.

The current date which the computer believes it to be will be shown in the lower-right corner of the screen. You should glance at this date on a regular basis during this program to insure that you are entering data on the correct date.

New Practice/Open Practice

First we need to start by creating the practice we will be working with. MediSoft allows you to store a number of practices in different areas, thus allowing you to only work on the billing of one practice at a time and prevents the billing of separate providers from becoming mixed.

It is important to open the practice at the beginning of each session or you will not be able to locate the patients, transactions, and other items which have been entered.

If you are doing billing for more than one practice (i.e., you work for a billing service which bills for numerous practices) it is important that you close one practice, and open the correct practice before switching from one practice to another. If you do not do so, you may enter data into the wrong practice. To switch from one practice to another, click on **File**, then on **Open Practice**. Next, choose the specific practice you wish to work on.

Open Practice allows you to access any of the practices which have been previously entered. Once you have created the CHS practice, you will use the **Open Practice** option to access its information.

Practice Information/Billing Information

The information contained in these screens will show up on various reports throughout the program, so it is important to insure that the information is complete and correct.

Practice Information is where you enter information about the actual provider of services. Billing Information is where you enter information about the Billing Service that handles billing for that provider. Since CHS does its own billing, the billing information screen should be left blank.

Both the practice and billing information screens include the same fields. The information contained in these screens includes:

Practice/Billing Name: The name of the office. If you are working for an individual provider, the provider's name may go in this field. You may enter up to 30 characters (either letters, punctuation, or spaces).

Street: The street address of the office or provider. You may enter up to 30 characters. If abbreviation is needed, be sure that the information given on the line is sufficient to allow mail to be properly delivered.

A second street line has been created to allow you to enter additional data. This could be a suite number or a department to which items should be addressed (i.e., Billing Department).

Exercise 4 – 2: For this class, you will be working for Consolidated Health Services. To enter its practice information, click on the **File** menu option, then choose **New Practice.** Enter "Consolidated Health Services," choose a data path, and click **Create**.

To prevent your data from being corrupted by others using MediSoft on your computer, the practice name and data path should include your name. For example: Practice: Consolidated Health Services Mary. Data Path: C:\MediSoft\CHSMary.

A Practice Information screen will open. As you read through the descriptions of the following fields, enter the following information on your screen. Entries and corrections are made by pressing Tab until you reach the field in which you wish to enter or change data. You may also use your mouse to position the arrow in the correct field, and then click the left button. Once you have highlighted the field, type in the correct information and press Tab to move to the next field.

Enter the following information:

Practice Name: Consolidated Health Services (your name)
Street: 1357 Castle Blvd.
Suite 515
City: Colter
State: CO
Zip Code: 81222
Phone: (790) 555-4567
Fax Phone: (790) 555-6789
Type: Medical
Federal Tax ID: 80-1234567

When you have entered all data, be sure to save your changes by clicking on the **Save** box or by pressing **F3**. This will save the information to the database. Neglecting to do so will cause the data entered to be lost.

City: The city of the provider/biller. You may enter up to 20 characters.

State: The state in which the provider/biller practices. This should coincide with the official postal two-letter state abbreviation.

Zip Code: The provider's/biller's zip code. If the complete nine-digit zip code is known, enter the first five digits, a hyphen, and the remaining four digits.

Phone: The provider's phone number. The area code and phone number should be entered without parentheses or hyphens separating the numbers. The computer will automatically enter these marks where needed.

Extension: The phone extension of the office.

Fax Phone: The provider's/biller's fax phone number. The area code and phone number should be entered without parentheses or hyphens separating the numbers. The computer will automatically enter these marks where needed.

Type: MediSoft can be used by medical practices, anesthesiologists, chiropractors, and many other health care providers. Choose Medical, Anesthesia, or Chiropractic. If you are billing for several types of practitioners, this field should be reset to reflect the types of claims you are currently entering. Choosing Anesthesia will allow anesthesia minutes to be entered onto claims. Choosing Chiropractic will add a field for "Level of Subluxation." Consolidated Health Services is a medical provider, so you should choose **Medical**. However, there may be a few times you need to enter anesthesia claims. At that time you should reset the practice type to Anesthesia.

Federal Tax I.D.: Enter the tax ID number for the practice. This can be either an employer identification number (EIN) or a social security number (SSN for an individual provider practice).

Because this number may take either form, hyphens should be entered in the appropriate places.

Extra 1:/Extra 2: These fields allow for entry of additional information that is important.

Program Options

There are a couple of program options that should be checked before we proceed with the entry of codes, patients, and charges. These include a couple of the default settings which appear in the program.
1. Choose **File**.
2. Choose **Program Options**.

This brings up the program options which have been entered. There are four pages of program options: General, Data Entry, Aging Reports, and HIPAA.

The **General** options include reminding you to back up your data before exiting the program and the windows which will appear on the screen as you start up the program. We will not be changing the settings on this page.

To get to the Data Entry options, click on the **Data Entry** tab or press **E**.

You do want to use "**Enter to move between the fields**", and to "**Force Payments To Be Applied**", so be sure there is a √ in the box to the left of these choices. These boxes are toggle (on/off) switches. Thus, clicking once on either the box or the words next to the box will turn the item on. Clicking it again will turn it off. The √ indicates the item is turned on.

You also want the computer to "Multiply units times amount", so be sure there is a √ in the box to the left of this choice. When entering transaction entries, it is possible to indicate that a procedure was performed several times or for several days by entering an appropriate number in the days or units field. A √ in this box will tell the computer to multiply the number of days or units by the charge for this service. Thus, if a doctor performs a minimal hospital visit on a patient two times over two days, the computer will show an extended charge of $200 total instead of the normal $100 per visit charge.

Default Place of Service: Entering a location code in this field will automatically print this default code as the location of services on the Transaction Entry screen. These codes correspond to the two-digit place of service (location) codes used in item 24B of the CMS-1500 Billing Form. The most common locations are:

11 Office
21 Inpatient Hospital
22 Outpatient Hospital
23 Emergency Room

For a complete list of codes, see instructions for completing a CMS-1500 Billing form, or the back of some CMS-1500 forms.

Once a default code is entered it will appear on every transaction entry charge. If the default location code is incorrect for the service provided, it may be changed by simply typing in a new location code. Since most of our billing will be for a medical office, we will use 11 as the default code.

To get to the Aging Reports options, click on the **Aging Reports** tab or press **A**.

Select the date and column parameters your office wishes to use when printing Patient or Insurance Aging Reports.

To get to the HIPAA options, click on the **HIPAA** tab or press **I**.

With the new privacy laws, it is essential that practices protect their data from unauthorized use or viewing. This function automatically logs off the program if there has been no activity for a set period of time. Basically, this option will shut off your computer if you stop using it or walk away from it. To get back into the program you will need to reenter the security code, if one is required for your office.

Once you have entered the desired information, exit the Program Options Screen by clicking on **Save** or by pressing the **F3** function key.

Remaining Options

The remaining options on the File screen will not be used at this time. However, in order to familiarize you with their functions, please read the information below.

Convert Data

In earlier versions, the Convert Data option allowed you to upgrade your software from a DOS to a Windows version of MediSoft. This function will take the information which a practice has stored in a MediSoft DOS format and convert it to a MediSoft Windows format so that it can be accessed by the windows program. This option does not appear on the more current versions of MediSoft.

Backup Data

The MediSoft program will warn you to back up your data prior to exiting the program and/or beginning a month-end processing. MediSoft assumes that your data is stored on the hard drive. When you back up your data, it will take the information which is stored on your hard drive and enter it onto the floppy disk in drive A (or D if you choose).

When information is stored on the hard drive of a computer, it can be accessed by anyone who uses that computer. Additionally, anyone who enters data will have it added to any data that was previously entered.

Discuss with your instructor whether or not you will be backing up files during this course. Your instructor may wish to have you back up files to a diskette, or to a secondary file on the hard drive.

Backup Data Files

Backing up your files is a safety precaution which actually saves your data to a second file or to a disk. Then if one file has a problem, you have the information stored in a second place.

MediSoft compresses the data at the time of backup to allow you to store more information on the files.

Destination Path: Enter the file or drive which holds your backup disk. Be sure that your disks have been formatted and inserted in the appropriate drive before answering this question. It may take more than one disk to backup your files. If so, the MediSoft system will prompt you when to insert a new diskette. The screen will tell you how much of the backup process is completed. It is important not to shut off the computer during the backup process as it could corrupt your data files.

Existing Backup Files: This field will show you the backup files which currently exist on the data path or drive you have chosen. This helps prevent you from copying over backup files you may need.

Password: If the security option requires that a password be entered to back up data, the password would be entered here. Not all practices will require a password to backup data. However, using a password insures that unauthorized persons are not able to make a copy of your patient files.

View Backup Disks

This option allows you to view the contents of a disk to be sure that the data was actually recorded to the backup disk.

Restore Data

This option allows you to restore (put back) information onto your hard drive that was either lost or corrupted. In order for this option to work, you must have a current backup copy of the data.

Be sure that you wish to restore the data as performing this function will cause all MediSoft information on your hard drive to be erased and replaced with the MediSoft data on the data diskette or backup file. Insert your backup disk into the proper disk drive, and then follow the instructions on the screen.

Security Setup

This option allows you to enter information on those people who are authorized to use the MediSoft system. It will also allow you to limit their access to certain files or commands.

File Maintenance

Choosing this option allows you to restore and rebuild your data files. This enables you to preserve the data and prevents you from having to reenter everything should a problem with your data files occur.

Also included in this menu option is the ability to purge (erase) information and recalculate patient balances.

Rebuild Indexes

This option allows you to rebuild the index files when they become damaged. If index files are not damaged, this procedure is not necessary since MediSoft automatically maintains all index files. However, it is recommended that you rebuild all indexes prior to doing the month-end processing. This will insure that all indexes are in a clean, undamaged state. Choose the index file(s) you wish to rebuild.

Rebuilding indexes can take a long time, depending on the amount of data contained in the indexes. Be sure to allow appropriate time. One of the best times to rebuild data indexes is to choose Rebuild All Files/Indexes just prior to leaving work for the night. Interruptions (power failures or surges, etc.) will not cause irreparable damage as the old index files are not deleted until the rebuilding has been completed.

Pack Data

In MediSoft, as in many computer programs, information that has been deleted is not actually erased from the file. It is simply marked as deleted, and the computer reuses that space when it needs to by recording new data over the old. This is similar to recording over previous messages on an answering machine or tape recorder rather than erasing the messages and then taping a new message over the blank tape.

This option allows you to erase the deleted data, thus condensing the amount of data in your files and increasing the amount of free storage space on your disk. To use this option, choose the file(s) you wish to purge (erase) deleted data from.

You should backup your data prior to using this function, just in case data has been inadvertently deleted from the system. When ready to proceed, be sure you have enough available disk space to complete the operation.

Recalculate Balances

This option allows you to recalculate and update patient balances and reset the date and amount of the last payment made by each patient. Recalculating balances updates the patient reference balances. These balances are used on the ledger window, walkout receipts, day sheets, and superbills.

If you wish to recalculate a single patient's balance information, this can be done in the Transaction Screen by clicking on the Account Total amount.

Purge Data

This option allows you to erase data from your data files, thus condensing the amount of data in your files and increasing the amount of free storage space on your disk. To use this option, choose the file(s) you wish to purge (erase).

Your choices include:
- Appointment Purge
- Claim Purge
- Statement Purge
- Recall Purge
- Purge Closed Cases
- Credit Card Purge

To use this option, click on one of the above choices, and then enter a cutoff date (for the first four items). All data in that file before **and including** the date specified will be deleted. Thus, if you choose Appointment Purge and enter a date of 1/1/XX, all appointments which had been entered for dates prior to and including 1/1/XX will be deleted.

Before a claim can be deleted using this system, it must be marked "Done." Therefore, it must have been printed, billed, and paid (or adjusted out). Claims which have a remaining balance due will not be purged.

You also have the option of purging **all closed cases**. By selecting this option, all closed cases will be purged, regardless of whether there is an outstanding balance or not. (For further information on "cases," see the Transaction Entry chapter of this text.)

You can also purge **Credit Card Entries**. Only credit card entries that are inactive are purged from the program. All credit card entries that are purged are recorded in the audit file. Purging removes the credit card entry number from the transaction file.

You should backup your data prior to using this function, just in case data has been inadvertently deleted from the system. When ready to proceed, be sure you have enough available disk space to complete the operation.

Summary

The File Menu options allow you to enter information pertaining to the practice, change the date, and choose default data. It also allows you to backup and restore data, and contains the File Maintenance option. The File Maintenance menu option allows you to rebuild your data files, recalculate balances, and purge data.

Questions for Review

Directions: Answer the following questions without looking back into the material just covered. Write your answers in the space provided.

1. What is the importance of ensuring that the practice information is correct before performing any transactions? _____

    _____

    _____

    _____

    _____

2. What three practice types are available in the Practice Information option screen?

    1. _____

    2. _____

    3. _____

3. What is the function of the Pack Data option? _____

    _____

    _____

4. What is the function of the Restore Data option? _____

    _____

5. What does it mean to Purge Data from your files? _____

    _____

    _____

    _____

If you were unable to answer any of the questions, refer back to that section, and then fill in the answers.

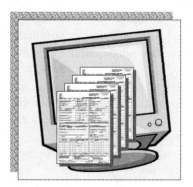

5

Lists Menu Options

After completion of this chapter you will be able to:

- Search for and delete an entry.
- Enter information in the Insurance Carrier List, Address List, Provider List, Referring Provider List, EDI/EMC Receivers List, Billing Code List, Procedure/Payment/Adjustment List, MultiLink List, and Diagnosis List.

Before you can enter transactions and create claims you will need to have some basic data entered into the computer. This data includes CPT® and ICD-9 codes, patient and insurance information, MultiLink codes, addresses, and provider information.

Because many of the other lists are accessed when entering patient data (Patients/Guarantors and Cases), we will discuss the completion of the other screens first. Completing the patient data screens will be discussed in Chapter 6.

Searching for an Entry

Upon entering most of the following screens, you will be automatically brought into the search screen. A listing of the previously entered entities (insurance carriers, addresses, providers, etc.) will appear in the middle of the screen. Highlight (click on) the entry you wish to access, and then choose Edit at the bottom of the screen.

If the entity you wish to work on is not shown in the search screen, you must search for it. To search for a specific entry in the 2004 version, first choose whether you wish to look for it under the code listing or by name (Different lists may have additional search options. For example, description, type, etc.). Make this selection in the **Field:** field by clicking on the "down arrow" on the top-right side of the screen. It is usually easiest to sort by name, since the code is not always known. To specify your preferred search parameters, click on the magnifying glass icon or down arrow (↓) to the right of the **Search for:** field.

As you enter a code or name in the **Search for:** field, the list in the lower part of the screen will automatically show all matching records. The more characters entered into the field, the more specific and narrow your search results will be. If there are no matches, the list will be blank. If there are several matches, you will be given a list of choices. Highlight the appropriate choice by clicking on it and clicking Edit. That entity's name and information will then appear on the screen.

To conduct a search in previous versions of MediSoft, click on the ↓ to the right of the **Sort By:** field. This will bring up the choice of sorting by code or by name.

Then move the cursor to the search field by clicking on the box to the right of Search. Enter a portion of the entity's name (i.e., Bal for Ball Insurance), then press enter. If there are no matches, you will hear a beep. If there is only one match, that entity's information will appear on the screen. If there are several matches, you will be given a list of choices. Click on the appropriate choice and press enter. That entity's name and information will then appear on the screen.

If you wish to enter a new entity, click on the "New" box at the bottom of the screen, or press **F8**.

Deleting an Entry

To delete an entity from any of the following lists, search for the entity using the search screen. Once found, highlight the entity's name on the screen, then hit the Delete key, or click on the Delete box at the bottom of the screen. You will be asked: "Are you sure you want to delete this record?" If so, click on "Yes" and the record will be deleted.

EDI/EMC Receivers List

Since information in the EDI/EMC Receivers List is used in several of the remaining lists, we will discuss it first.

With today's new technology, providers have the ability to transmit claims from their computers through phone lines and directly into another computer. The 2004 version of MediSoft calls this an electronic data interchange (EDI). In earlier versions of MediSoft, claims sent in this manner are called electronic media claims (EMC). Claims printed on paper and sent through the regular mail system are often called paper claims.

Electronic vs. Paper Claims
Electronic media claims have certain advantages over paper claims:
1. They take less time to submit, since they are transmitted directly through phone lines. There is no need to wait several days for them to be sent through the mail.
2. They use less paper and other supplies.
3. There is less of a chance that they will be lost or misplaced.
4. They are processed much more quickly (an average of about 10-15 days rather than the normal 30 days for paper claims).
5. There is less chance for error since the information does not need to be re-entered into the insurance carrier's computer.

6. There is less chance of the claim being rejected since it often goes through a clearinghouse which will do a preliminary check to make sure all required fields are completed.
7. It lowers costs, requiring less personnel time for printing and mailing the claims, and for entering the data in the insurance carrier computers.
8. It saves time for the provider since each claim does not need to be signed. The provider's signature on the agreement between the insurance carrier and the provider is considered valid for all claims submitted electronically.

Direct Submission vs. Clearinghouse
When claims are submitted electronically, they are sent through the phone lines using a modem. Some carriers allow you to submit claims directly to them, but many others prefer that the claims are first sent to a clearinghouse. The claims are then checked by the clearinghouse to be sure that all of the necessary information has been completed on the claim and there are no glaring errors (i.e., female procedure performed on a male patient, procedures with no relationship to the given diagnosis, etc.). Once checked, the claims are then sent on to the insurance carrier.

Using a clearinghouse allows the carrier to reject fewer claims, since those which are not complete or have glaring errors are never submitted to them. It saves personnel time as well as resources that might be spent contacting the provider for further information.

Submitting Claims Using MediSoft
The MediSoft system allows you to submit claims electronically either through a clearinghouse or directly to a carrier. Once all the data has been entered through the appropriate screens, claims can be generated and sent using the Claim Management screen.

Training facilities cannot submit electronic claims because they have not been assigned appropriate clearinghouse codes and to go through the process of submitting a claim electronically would actually send the claim out. Additionally, trying to send out claims when your computer is not properly hooked up to phone lines could cause some of your data to be lost. For that reason, CHS will submit all claims on paper. However, a preliminary relationship with a clearinghouse has been established, so we will enter the data we currently have on them.

The first step to creating electronic data interchange/electronic media claims is to enter the information regarding the company which will be receiving the claims. This can be either the insurance carrier directly, or a clearinghouse.

Exercise 5 – 1: CHS will be submitting claims through a clearinghouse. In the Lists menu, click on EDI/EMC Receivers. At the bottom of the screen, click New. Enter the following information for the clearinghouse:

Name: EDI Always
Address: 4123 Media Blvd.
Colter, CO 81225
Phone: (800) 555-3452 X456
Fax: (800) 555-6789
Contact: Emily Encoder
Data Phone: (800) 555-3746
Submitter ID: CHSAA123
Password: CHS0001

There are three screens in the EDI/EMC Receiver List: the Address, Modem, and ID and Extra screens.

Address Screen

Code: The computer will automatically assign an access code for each address entered, or you can enter a code yourself. Codes may contain letters or numbers and can be up to five characters.

Name: Enter the name of the EDI/EMC receiving company. You have up to 30 characters.

Street: Enter the street address of the EDI/EMC receiving company. Two lines are provided to allow for a complete address.

City: Enter the city of the EDI/EMC receiving company.

State: Enter the state of the EDI/EMC receiving company. This should correspond with the two letter postal code for a state.

Zip Code: Enter the zip code of the EDI/EMC receiving company. If the complete nine digit zip code is known, enter the first five digits, a hyphen, and the remaining four digits.

Phone: Enter the EDI/EMC receiving company's phone number. This should be the number you can call and reach a person, not the number which your computer/modem should call to connect with their computer/modem. No hyphens or parentheses are needed. The computer will automatically enter these.

Fax: Enter the EDI/EMC receiving company's fax number. No hyphens or parentheses are needed. The computer will automatically enter these.

Contact: Enter your contact within the EDI/EMC receiving company. This can be either a person or a department.

Comment: Enter any comments regarding the EDI/EMC receiving company. These can be items such as the best time to call them, their hours or other pertinent information.

Modem Screen

Data Phone: Enter the phone number which your modem should call to reach their modem. This is often different from the regular phone number.

Dialing Prefix: Enter any prefix needed for dialing this number. If this is an international number, enter the country code.

Dialing Suffix: Enter any suffix needed for dialing this number.

Serial Port/Parity/Baud Rate/Data Bits/ Transmit Protocol/Stop Bits: This is information detailing the type of modem you have and how it sends information (speed, etc.). This information should appear automatically if your computer is already connected to a modem. If not, you will need to consult the manual for your specific type of modem for the correct data to enter here.

Modem Initialization: This field is normally left blank. It is used only when you are having difficulties with the program not "hanging up" after the transmission. You may also need this option if the modem is required to be left in a certain state (i.e., Auto Answer mode).

Modem Termination: Some modems require a string of characters to modify the modem that the transmission is complete and the call should be terminated. Your modem instruction manual will tell you if this applies to your modem. In most cases this field is left blank.

Dialing Attempt: Enter the number of attempts you want your computer to make before abandoning the attempt to send information. If this field is left blank, the program will make up to 99 dialing attempts.

Transmission Mode: You have two choices for this setting. Test is used if you are not actively sending a claim, but merely want to test if the EDI/EMC receiver is properly receiving your transmission. Active is used if you are actually sending a claim. For this class, this field should always be set to Test.

ID and Extra Screen
Submitter ID 1 and 2: This is a code which will be given to the practice by the EDI/EMC receiver. It allows the EDI/EMC receiver to identify who is sending the claims. It is similar to an account number. MediSoft allows up to two submitter IDs for each EDI/EMC receiver.

Submitter Password 1 and 2: This field is for entering the password to submit claims. This is similar to having a password at the bank before your account can be accessed. It is a security precaution to insure that others do not submit claims using your account number, since clearinghouses often charge by the number of claims submitted.

Program File: This is a number given to you by your EDI/EMC receiver.

Extra 1 through 6: These fields are for entering additional data which is needed to submit claims to this EDI/EMC receiver. The data to be entered in these fields will often be assigned by the EDI/EMC receiver.

File Name ID: This is a field which allows MediSoft to communicate by modem with the

MediSoft clearinghouse. This field should not be changed unless you are instructed to do so by MediSoft.

Be sure to save your data before exiting this screen.

Insurance Carrier List

To access the Insurance Carrier List, click on the Insurance Carrier List icon, or choose the **Lists** Menu option and choose **Insurance Carriers**.

This option allows you to see and enter information regarding a patient's insurance carrier. This includes not only the name and address for the insurance carrier, but also the insurance type and information on how the carrier prefers to have forms printed.

To enter a new insurance carrier, click New at the bottom of the screen or press the **F8** function key. To edit the information of an insurance carrier that is already entered, click on the carrier in the list and click Edit at the bottom of the screen or press the **F9** function key.

When creating or editing insurance carrier information, you will input information into various screens. The 2004 version of MediSoft includes Address, Options, EDI Codes, and PINs screens. Earlier versions of the software have only Address, Options, and EMC Codes screens.

Exercise 5 – 2: Sue Pervisor gives you the patient information sheets for the Dunnitt and Waite families (Document 1 and 2 from Section 4). While going through the instructions for each screen, enter the insurance carrier data for these families.

Address Screen
The address screen allows you to enter name, address, and phone information of an insurance carrier.

Code: The computer will automatically assign a code for each carrier entered. If desired, you may assign a code. This can be a series of numbers or letters. Some practices will choose to enter the first five characters of the insurance carrier's name. If those numbers have already been used, then enter the first four characters followed by a number (i.e., Winter Insurance would be Winte, Wintell Insurers would be Wint1, etc.).

Name: Enter the name of the insurance carrier. This field must be completed or you will not be allowed to save this carrier.

Street: Enter the street address of the insurance carrier. You have two lines to enter their complete address. If mail is to be addressed to a specific department (i.e., Attn: Claims Dept.) that information can be placed on the first line with the street address given on the following line.

City: Enter the city in which the insurance carrier is located.

State: Enter the state in which the insurance carrier is located. This should coincide with the official postal two-letter state abbreviation.

Zip Code: Enter the insurance carrier's zip code. If the complete nine-digit zip code is known, enter the first five digits, a hyphen, and the remaining four digits.

Phone: Enter the insurance carrier's phone number. Do not add hyphens or parentheses, the computer will automatically put these in.

Extension: Enter the extension for the insurance carrier. This will often be the extension for the claims department, since they are the department which is most often contacted by a provider.

Fax: Enter the insurance carrier's fax phone number. Do not add hyphens or parentheses.

Contact: Enter the name of your contact at the insurance carrier, if known. This can be a specific person who handles your accounts or the name of a department.

Practice ID Number: Many insurance carriers, especially HMOs and PPOs assign a number to the practice to help identify it. If applicable, enter that number here.

Options Screen

To get to the Options screen, simply click on the word **Options** at the top of the Insurance Carrier List screen.

Plan Name: Enter the plan name assigned by the insurance carrier. This allows the insurance carrier to more readily access the proper contract or policy. This information corresponds with box 9d or 11c on a CMS-1500.

Type: This item will indicate the type of claim being submitted to this carrier. Click on the ↓ arrow to the right of the Type: field to bring up a complete list of insurance carrier types. To choose a type, simply click on the type desired.

Bring up the list of insurance carrier types, and then look at a CMS-1500 form. If one of the first seven Type codes is chosen, where will this information show up on a CMS-1500 claim form?

Procedure Code Set: It is possible to enter up to three procedure codes for a given procedure. This is most often used with Medicare HCPCS codes and with states or carriers which have their own coding system. The CPT® code should be entered in the first procedure code box, then the corresponding HCPCS or state procedure code entered into the second and third code fields. By entering a 1, 2, or 3, MediSoft knows which set of codes to use when billing this carrier. For this class, if no code set is indicated on your paperwork, enter 1 to print CPT® codes. If this is for a Medicare claim, enter 2 to indicate the use of HCPCS codes.

Diagnosis Code Set: Likewise, it is possible to enter up to three diagnosis codes for a given diagnosis. This is most often used with states or carriers which have their own coding system. The ICD-9 code should be entered in the first diagnosis code box, then the corresponding state diagnosis code entered into the second and third code fields. By entering a 1, 2, or 3, MediSoft knows which set of codes to use when billing this carrier. For this class, enter 1 to print ICD-9 codes.

Patient Signature on File/Insured Signature on File/Physician Signature on File: Different carriers occasionally prefer to have different items printed in the signature boxes of the CMS-1500 (items 12, 13, and 31). Click on the ↓ to the right of each Signature on File field. If this carrier wishes the words "Signature on File" to print in the CMS-1500 signature boxes, click on that option. To print the name of the patient and/or insured in items 12 and 13 and the name of the provider in item 31, click on the Print Name option. If you wish nothing to print in items 12, 13, and 31, click on Leave Blank. If nothing is printed in the boxes, the patient will need to sign items 12 and 13 and the provider will need to sign item 31 before the claim can be submitted.

While these boxes will determine what the carrier wishes to have printed in the box ("Signature on File," the patient's/insured's/physician's name, or nothing), the patient and the physician have the right to determine whether or not they agree to the provisions listed in these boxes. The patient must have previously signed an authorization to release information and an assignment of benefits. If these documents are not signed, then nothing should be printed in these boxes. For that reason, the patient information file in the Patient/Guarantor List (see Chapter 6) has a box to indicate whether or not these items have been signed. Therefore, the patient record actually controls whether anything will be placed in these boxes. This box only allows the carrier to determine what wording they prefer to have written in these boxes if the permission has been granted.

Likewise, the provider information screen in the Provider List allows the provider to make the determination of whether the computer will sign the form for him (using "Signature on File" or the provider's name), or whether the item will be left blank.

For this class, all insurance carriers should have nothing placed in the signature boxes. The biller should sign each CMS-1500 as the provider representative.

Print PINs on Forms: Occasionally, services rendered in a provider's office will be rendered by staff other than the provider himself. Medicare and Medicaid require that, if the provider rendering services is not the attending provider (the one listed in item 33 of the CMS-1500), that the provider who rendered each service be identified in box 24K of the CMS-1500.

This box allows you the option of printing the provider's name and PIN, the PIN only, or to leave the area blank. For this class, leave the area blank.

Default Billing Method: This box allows you to choose whether this carrier prefers to have claims submitted electronically or on paper. By clicking on the ↓ to the right of this field, you can choose either Paper or Electronic. For this class, we will be printing all claims on paper. If a carrier has agreed to accept electronic claims from this provider, choosing Electronic in this box will instruct the computer not to print these claims on paper, but to send them electronically.

EDI/EMC Codes Screen

The third screen is for entering information for submitting electronic media claims (EMC) to this carrier.

EDI/EMC Receiver: Enter the code for the EDI/EMC receiver (the company or organization which will receive your EDI/EMC claims for this carrier). In order for an EDI/EMC carrier to have a code, they must have previously been entered under the EDI/EMC Receivers List (see **List, EDI/EMC Receivers**). You may search for an EDI/EMC Receiver's code by clicking on the magnifying glass to the right of this field or by pressing **F6**. If the EDI/EMC Receiver has not been previously entered, press **F8** to add it to the EDI/EMC Receiver List.

EDI/EMC Payor/EDI/EMC Sub-ID/NDC Record Code: These entry fields will be assigned to you by the Electronic Claims Submission company which handles your claims. They are used for identification purposes.

EDI/EMC Extra 1/Medigap/EDI/EMC Extra 2: These fields are for entering extra information regarding EDI/EMC claims for this carrier. They are often not used.

EDI Max Transactions: Some carriers will limit the number of claims that can be submitted at one time. Enter the maximum number of claims allowed by each carrier. Often this field is left blank.

After entering insurance carrier data, be sure to hit **F3** to save, or click on the **Save** button. The insurance carrier will then be added to the Insurance Carrier List which will appear on the screen.

To exit the insurance carrier screen, click on the **Close** button.

Address List

This section of the MediSoft system is used as an address file to hold the names, addresses, and phone numbers which your practice needs. The MediSoft system also uses this section to store data on a patient's employer. Other pertinent addresses may include referring physicians, facilities, or attorneys.

To access the Address List, click on the Address List icon, or choose the **Lists** Menu option and click **Addresses**.

Exercise 5 – 3: While reading through this screen, enter the pertinent information regarding place of employment for D. Jobb Dunnitt and Hugh Waite (Documents 1 and 2). Click New to enter information.

Code: The computer will automatically assign an access number for each address entered or you can enter a code yourself. Codes may contain letters or numbers and can be up to five characters.

Name: Enter the name of the person, employer, facility, etc.

Street: Enter the street address for the addressee.

City: Enter the city for the addressee.

State: Enter the state for the addressee. This should coincide with the official postal two-letter state abbreviation.

Zip Code: Enter the addressee's zip code. If the complete nine-digit zip code is known, enter the first five digits, a hyphen, and the remaining four digits.

Type: This field allows you to differentiate between the types of addresses listed. MediSoft has six types of address records:
- Attorney,
- Employer,
- Facility*,
- Laboratory,
- Miscellaneous, and
- Referral Source.

*A facility address can be any type of medical facility, including a hospital, urgent care facility, rest home, etc.

Phone: Enter the addressee's phone number. Do not use parentheses or hyphens.

Extension: Enter the extension for the addressee.

Fax Phone: Enter the addressee's fax phone number. Do not use parentheses or hyphens.

Cell Phone: Enter the addressee's personal cell phone number. Do not use parentheses or hyphens.

Office: Enter the addressee's office number, or the number at which they can be reached at work. Do not use parentheses or hyphens.

Contact: Enter the name of the contact person for the addressee if one is known.

E-Mail: Enter the addressee's e-mail address.

ID: Enter the UPIN number for referring providers. This number will then print in the required box on the CMS-1500 (item 17a).

Identifier: Enter the Employer Identification Number (EIN) for the addressee. This is a HIPAA-compliance field.

Extra 1/Extra 2: Enter additional data regarding the person or entity listed above.

Provider List

This screen is for entering information about the providers in the practice. Additional practice staff (i.e., nurses, billers, etc.) may also be entered in this file.

To access the Provider List, click on the Provider List icon, or choose the **Lists** Menu option and choose **Providers**.

Exercise 5 – 4: Since the MediSoft system is new to CHS, none of the providers have been entered into the system. Take out the Provider Information List (Document 3). While going through the following descriptions, enter the information for the CHS doctors.

In the 2004 version of MediSoft, there are four information screens in the Provider List: Address, Default Pins, Default Group IDs, and PINs. In earlier versions there are just two screens in the Provider List: the Address screen and the PINs and IDs screen.

Address Screen

Code: The computer will automatically assign an access code for each provider entered, or you can enter a code yourself. Codes may contain letters or numbers and can be up to five characters. Up to 99 providers may be entered in this file. (NOTE: If MediSoft assigns the code, it will often use the provider's initials.) Once a code has been assigned, it may not be changed.

Inactive: Check this box if you need to deactivate a provider, but not delete him/her. This may need to be done if a provider is no longer with the practice, but all the claims have not yet been paid. If there are still open issues on the claims of this provider, the provider needs to remain in the system. Placing a provider on inactive status may prevent you from entering new claims for this provider.

Last Name: Enter the last name of the provider. You have up to 20 characters. If the name is longer than 20 characters, most providers will prefer you to type in the name as it appears, until you run out of space. This will allow names to be alphabetized more correctly than if you attempt to abbreviate the name by leaving out letters in the middle of the name.

Middle Initial: Enter the middle initial of the provider.

First Name: Enter the first name of the provider.

Credentials: Enter the provider's credentials. This will normally be M.D.

Street: Enter the street address of the provider. Two lines are provided to allow for a complete address.

City: Enter the provider's city.

State: Enter the provider's state. This should correspond with the two-letter postal code for a state.

Zip Code: Enter the provider's zip code. If the complete nine-digit zip code is known, enter the first five digits, a hyphen, and the remaining four digits.

E-Mail: Enter the provider's e-mail address.

Office: Enter the provider's office phone number. No hyphens or parentheses are needed.

Fax: Enter the provider's fax number. No hyphens or parentheses are needed.

Home: Enter the provider's home phone number. No hyphens or parentheses are needed.

Cell: Enter the provider's personal cell phone number. No parentheses or hyphens are needed.

Signature on File: This box determines whether the computer will print "Signature on File" or the physician's name, in item 31 of the CMS-1500. This is an on/off choice. By clicking on this option, it will place an X in the box if there is not one, or remove the X if there is one. If an X is placed in the box, the Signature Date field will be highlighted to allow you to enter the date which the provider's signature was placed on file. CHS requires all claims to be signed by the provider or the provider's representative (you). Therefore nothing should be printed in this field. You should sign and date all claims.

Medicare Participating: Many providers sign agreements with Medicare for treating Medicare patients. Among other things, this agreement limits the amount which the provider can accept for payment of services to Medicare patients. If the provider accepts Medicare assignment, enter an X in this box. If not, leave it blank.

License Number: Each state licenses providers to practice in that state. Enter the provider's state license number.

Specialty: Indicate the provider's specialty. For a complete list of specialties, click on the ↓ to the right of the field. Then choose a specialty by clicking on the appropriate specialty for the provider.

Default PINs Screen

SSN/Federal Tax ID: All persons and companies are required to have a tax ID number. For individuals, this is a social security number (SSN). For companies, it is an employer identification number (EIN). Enter the tax ID number here, including hyphens in the appropriate places, and indicate whether this is an SSN or EIN in the toggle boxes to the right.

Medicare PIN: This field is for a single provider's Medicare assigned PIN.

Medicaid PIN/Medicare PIN/Blue Cross/Blue Shield PIN/Commercial PPO/HMO PIN: Medicaid, TRICARE/CHAMPUS, Blue Cross/Blue Shield, and some other commercial carriers may also use identifying numbers for their providers. Enter each that applies in the appropriate fields. When any of these fields, the Medicare PIN field or the UPIN field, are used, the computer will print the appropriate PIN number in item 33 of the CMS-1500.

PPO: If the provider is a member of a PPO network, enter the assigned PPO number here.

HMO: If the provider is a member of an HMO network, enter the assigned HMO number here.

UPIN: Enter the provider's Unique Physician Identifying Number (UPIN). When a provider orders services for a Medicare patient or refers a patient to another provider, this number is required.

Where does a referring provider's UPIN appear on a CMS-1500?

_____

Extra 1/Extra 2: Enter additional data regarding the person or entity listed above.

EDI/EMC ID: Providers are often assigned an identifying number for Electronic Media Claims (EMC). This number would be assigned by the EMC clearinghouse. We will not be using this number.

CLIA Number: This number is assigned to lab providers submitting electronic claims through NDC.

TAT Number: This number is assigned to providers submitting electronic claims through NDC.

National Identifier: This is a 15 digit alphanumeric identifier assigned by HCFA. It is required for HIPAA compliance.

Default Group IDs Screen

Group Number: Often a provider is part of a medical group. In such a case, Medicare may assign a group Provider Identification Number (PIN) rather than one PIN to each of the doctors. If this is the case, enter the group PIN number here. All CHS doctors have the same group PIN. It is CHS123.

Medicare Group ID: If the group has a Medicare assigned UPIN, enter that number here.

Medicaid Group ID: If the group has a Medicaid assigned UPIN, enter that number here.

BC/BS Group ID: If the group has a Blue Cross/Blue Shield assigned UPIN, enter that number here.

Other Group ID: If the group has any other assigned UPIN, enter that number here.

Where does a provider's group number appear on a CMS-1500?

_____

PINs Screen

This screen shows a list of entered providers' PINs and Group IDs for the various insurance carriers they interact with, and their corresponding codes.

After entering each provider's data, be sure to hit **F3** to save, or click on the **Save** button. The provider will then be added to the Provider List.

To exit the Provider screen, click on the **Close** button.

Referring Provider List

This list is for entering data on providers who have referred patients to the practice. It will be used to track referrals and to complete Items 17 and 17a on the CMS-1500.

These fields are the same as the fields for the Provider List. For instructions on completing these fields, see the above information.

Billing Code List

Often practices split their billing into several groups. This allows for continuous income during the month, as well as prevents the major backlog of work which can happen with billing all patients at once. By using this field, you can place patients into groups for billing purposes. Patients can be grouped together by last name (i.e., A – M is billed on the first of the month and N – Z is billed on the 15th of the month), insurance carrier or type of insurance (i.e., Medicare, Medicaid, group insurance, etc.), or by various other methods.

The Billing Code List opens to a window with a list alphabetized by code of all previously entered billing codes. From this window you can search for existing information. To enter new codes click New at the bottom of the window.

Code: A two-digit alphanumeric code which identifies this billing code.

Description: A description of the billing code. For example, if you were to bill all patients with last names starting with A – M at one time, and all patients with last names starting with N – Z at

another time, your first code could be AM and the description Patient Names A – M.

Since we are using so few patients, we will bill them all at once. Therefore, you may leave this space blank.

Procedure/Payment/Adjustment List

This file is used to store data regarding all transactions which may be used in the Transaction Entry screen. These include not only CPT® codes, but also payments and adjustments which are necessary for keeping accurate accounting records. In reality, many providers purchase computerized CPT® lists which can be automatically loaded into the computer each year. The practice then adds its own codes for payments and adjustments.

To access the Procedure/Payment/Adjustment List, click on the CPT® icon, or choose the **Lists** Menu option and choose **Procedures/Payments/ Adjustments**.

This may be the one screen where it may be easier to sort by the code rather than the description, based on whether the CPT® code is known or not. Descriptions of medical terms can sometimes be confusing, and there are often numerous choices for the same type of procedure. For example, if you are searching for an office visit, you may end up with over ten choices depending upon whether the patient is new or established, and the complexity of the visit.

Exercise 5 – 5: Sue Pervisor gives you a list of procedures which have not yet been entered in the Procedure Code List (Document 4). Look up the proper procedure code in the CPT® and enter the procedures into the Procedures/Payments/ Adjustments screen. All items are charges and the accounting code should be given as 4010 for medicine charges, 4020 for surgery, 4030 for consultation, 4040 for diagnostic x-ray, 4050 for diagnostic lab, 4060 for radiation therapy, and 4070 for anesthesia.

When editing or creating new codes, there are two screens in the Procedure/Payment/Adjustment List; the General screen and the Amounts screen.

The General screen provides all the necessary information regarding the type of code, the description, and insurance printing information. The Amounts screen contains information regarding the charges for the procedure and the cost to the practice.

General Screen

Code 1: Enter the procedure code. This can be either an alphabetical or numerical code of up to ten characters. For CPT® codes, enter the five digit CPT® code. Alphabetic codes would be entered for other procedures. For example, to indicate a cash payment by the patient you could enter the code: CSHPMT.

Inactive: Check this box if you need to deactivate a code, but not delete it. This may need to be done if a CPT® code has been deleted by the AMA, but all previous claims with this code have not yet been paid. If there are still open issues on the claims, the code needs to remain in the system. Having a code on an inactive status may prevent you from entering this code on new claims.

Description: Enter a description of the procedure. Your entry space is limited. You are allowed up to 40 characters. When entering CPT® codes, be sure that all necessary information for choosing the correct CPT® code is entered in the description.

How would you abbreviate the following description: Office or outpatient visit with a problem-focused history and exam and straightforward medical decision making.
Write your description in the space provided below. Do not use more than 40 characters.

_____

_____

Code Type: The following is an alphabetized list of the code types which may be present, depending on your version of the MediSoft software. You must choose one of the following code types to identify the type of procedure.

    Adjustment. This code is used for adjustments to a charge. These can be anything such as a courtesy reduction of a patient's bill or a correction of an incorrect billing.

Billing Charge. These are normal charges used for billing.

Cash Copayment. If the patient pays their copayment by cash, this code should be used.

Cash Payment. The patient has made a cash payment on this account. This is for patients who make cash payments on the amount of the charges which are their responsibility.

Check Copayment. If the patient pays their copayment by check, this code should be used.

Check Payment. This code indicates that a patient has paid for services with a personal check.

Comment. This code allows a comment to be entered onto the patient's account.

Credit Card Copayment. If the patient pays their copayment by credit card, this code should be used.

Credit Card Payment. If the patient made a payment by credit card, this code should be used.

Deductible. Indicates that this is a payment made to cover the patient's deductible amount.

Inside Lab Charge. If there were charges for a lab contained within the facility, this code should be used.

Insurance Adjustment. The amount has been adjusted due to information from the insurance carrier.

Insurance Payment. The insurance carrier is making a payment on this account.

Insurance Take Back Adjustment. An adjustment made by an insurance carrier.

Insurance Withhold Adjustment. An amount withheld by an insurance carrier until the end of the year. This amount must be adjusted against the patient's account.

Medicare Adjustment. This adjustment is being made to write-off the difference between a billed charge and a Medicare approved amount.

Outside Lab Charge. The charges are for a lab not connected with this facility.

Procedure Charge. The service being performed will create a charge on the patient's account. A charge code would be used for all CPT® Codes and other services or procedures for which a patient is charged (i.e., missed appointment charge).

Product Charge. The charge is for a product rather than a procedure. For example, a person may require crutches to assist them with walking or a sling for a sprained wrist.

Tax. The charges are for tax. This is usually associated with a product charge.

The practice may type in any code they wish to indicate services, charges, adjustments, etc., for any of these procedures. For example, an entry with the Code MCRADJ and the code type of Adjustment, could be used to identify the amount above the Medicare approved amount which is being written off the patient's account. The practice may set up any number of procedure codes within a procedure type. Therefore, they can list several different types of adjustments, all with the Adjustment procedure type.

Account Code: Enter the four-digit general ledger account number which pertains to these services. This allows transactions to be categorized according to their type so that all similar charges, payments or adjustments may be grouped together on reports and in the company's accounting system.

Type of Service: A complete list of these codes will be provided by your carrier. These codes correspond to the general descriptions given in the CPT® and add in a few other types of services. A partial list includes:

1 – Medicine
2 – Surgery
3 – Consultation
4 – Diagnostic X-ray
5 – Diagnostic Lab
6 – Radiation Therapy
7 – Anesthesia
8 – Surgical Assistance
9 – Other Medical
0 – Blood Charges

Place of Service: Enter the two-digit code corresponding with the place where this service is normally performed (i.e., Office visits are done in an office). These codes correspond to the two-digit place of service (location) codes used in item 24B of the CMS-1500 Billing Form. The most common locations associated with medical billing are:

11 Office
21 Inpatient Hospital
22 Outpatient Hospital
23 Emergency Room

For a complete list of codes, see instructions for completing a CMS-1500 Billing form, or the back of the many CMS-1500 forms.

Once a code is entered here it will appear on every transaction entry charge. If the default location code is incorrect for the service provided, it may be changed by simply typing in a new location code.

Enter the appropriate code for each of the services you are entering.

Time to Do Procedure: Enter the amount of time it usually takes to perform the procedure. This information is used when scheduling appointments.

Alternate Codes 2/3: If an alternate coding system is used by one or more of the insurance carriers, the alternate codes for the procedure listed can be entered here. The computer can then automatically choose the correct code to enter on the billing form. For example, if the Code Number 2 slot is used for HCPCS codes and the Medicare carrier listed in the Insurance Information file has a 2 in the Procedure Code Type Set, then any HCPCS listed in this spot will automatically print on the billing form for the Medicare carrier.

Taxable: This indicates that the associated item is taxable.

Patient Only Responsible: An X in this box indicates that the patient only is responsible for these charges. Thus, these charges will not be billed to an insurance carrier, or show up on a claim form. They will, however, show up on a patient statement or walkout receipt. Examples of charges that may be patient only responsible include cosmetic services, experimental services, dietary services, or charges for a patient missing a scheduled appointment.

Don't Bill To Insurance/Don't Print On: If this procedure should not be charged for certain carriers, you can program the computer to print only for those carriers by inserting an insurance carrier number or a carrier type in this space. Carrier numbers should be separated by commas. For example, if Red is carrier #1, White #2, and Blue #3, and you want this procedure not to print on Red and Blue, then enter 1,3. If this procedure should print only on Medicare, Medicaid, and TRICARE/ CHAMPUS billings, enter MAC in this area. When entering Insurance Types, no comma is needed between the letter codes. (For further information on insurance types, see the Insurance Types field under Insurance Carrier List.)

Only Bill To Insurance/Only Print On Insurance: This field works the same as the above field, except that this procedure will print only on the carriers listed.

Default Modifiers: If there is a modifier normally associated with this code, enter the modifier here. This will automatically print the modifier on transactions involving this code. If the code is not correct for a given transaction, it may be deleted by simply typing over it.

HIPAA Approved: Checking this box indicates that this code is HIPAA approved.

Revenue Code: Enter the revenue code associated with this procedure. This is for use when billing UB-92 or hospital claims.

Default Units: Enter the common number of units associated with this procedure. This will most often be 1. If the code is not correct for a given transaction, it may be deleted by simply typing over it.

Purchased Service: Enter a check in the box if this procedure is a service purchased from another entity (i.e., a procedure done by an outside lab).

Amounts Screen

Charge Amounts A: Enter the standard charge for the procedure in this field. This charge will automatically show up when the procedure is entered into the Transaction Entry screen. If a different amount is to be charged for an individual customer, this default can always be overridden by simply typing in the new charge. Be aware that CHS has a standard charge for all procedures, but not all doctors in the CHS family will charge the same amount for the same procedures. Doctors set their own prices. Therefore, you should check the amount the provider chooses to bill when entering charges in the Transaction Entry screen. This

amount will be listed on the claims next to the description of the service.

Cost of Service/Product: Enter here the practice's cost of providing this service or their cost for a product. This can include the cost of outside lab services, or the cost of supplies and other items which are used in conjunction with this service (i.e., cotton swabs, tongue depressors, etc.). This field is optional and is used to help a practice establish how much they are actually making on the services provided.

Medicare Allowed Amount: Enter the amount allowed by Medicare for this procedure if you are a participating provider. If you are not a participating provider, enter the amount which you are allowed to bill Medicare patients for this procedure. This is usually the Medicare allowed amount plus 15% which you may balance bill the patient. This field helps to calculate any write-off between the standard billed amount and the Medicare Approved Amount.

After entering procedure, payment, or adjustment data, be sure to hit **F3** to save, or click on the Save button. Your information will then be added to the Procedure/Payment/Adjustment List which will appear on the screen.

To exit the Procedure/Payment/Adjustment screen, click on the **Close** button.

Exercise 5 – 6: Using the Procedure/Payment/ Adjustment List Screen located under the Lists function on the menu bar, input the procedure codes and Accounting codes for the descriptions given below.

Description	Procedure Code	Acctg Code
Patient Check Payment	PT CHECK	1020
Payment By Cash	CASH	1010
Insurance Payment	INS PMT	1030
Standard Adjustment	ADJ STD	1070
Insurance Adjustment	ADJ INS	1080
Check Copayment	COPAY CK	1060
Cash Copayment	COPAY CASH	1090
Inside Lab Charges	LAB IN	1110
Outside Lab Charges	LAB OUT	1100
Comment	COMMENT	No Code
Credit Card Payment	CREDIT PMT	1040

MultiLink List

When a certain diagnosis is suspected or confirmed, there are often a set of routine procedures which are all performed together. This screen allows the practice to enter a single code for the procedures which, when entered in the Transaction Entry screen, will list all the procedures. This eliminates having the biller enter each of the procedures one at a time. It also prevents a code from being inadvertently left off the list.

To enter the MultiLink List, click on the **Lists** menu option and choose **MultiLink Codes**.

Exercise 5 – 7: Allotta Payne M.D., OB-GYN has asked that the following information be entered into a MultiLink screen. These procedures are always performed together when a patient is pregnant. She has provided a description of the procedures, but is unsure of the proper CPT® codes for them. Look up the proper CPT® codes and then enter the data into the MultiLink Screen.

MultiLink Code: PREG

Description	CPT® Code
Office Visit, mod complexity	_____
Urinalysis	_____
Obstetric Lab Panel	_____

Code: Enter an alphabetical or numerical code for this MultiLink. The most helpful ones are those that will help you remember the description of what the MultiLink is for (i.e., DIABSCR for Diabetes Screening). If you do not wish to enter a code, the computer will assign one for you.

Description: Enter a description of the diagnosis or condition.

Link Code 1/2/3/4/5/6/7: Enter the procedure codes associated with this MultiLink. Each of the procedure codes must have been previously entered into the Procedure/Payment/Adjustment Codes List. If they have not been, you will need to add them before entering the codes here. If the codes have

been entered but you are unsure of the code, use **F6** or the magnifying glass icon to search for the procedure. To add a new code to the Procedure/Payments/Adjustment Code List without backing out of this screen, use the **F8** key.

Link Code #8: Enter the eighth code associated with this MultiLink. If more than eight codes are needed, enter the MultiLink code for an additional MultiLink. All procedures in this secondary MultiLink will then be added to the procedures listed above.

For example, let's say you want to enter a MultiLink for the procedures performed for an unexplained death, and there are ten separate procedures done (requiring ten separate codes). You would name the MultiLink code UNEXDTH. Then enter the first seven procedure codes in the fields for link codes 1 through 7. On link code number 8, you would enter UNEXDTH2. You then create a second MultiLink entry under the code UNEXDTH2 in which you will enter the remaining three codes on MultiLink codes 1 through 3. When the code UNEXDTH is entered into the Transaction Entry screen, it will automatically print all ten codes on separate lines on the Transaction Entry screen.

After entering MultiLink data, be sure to hit **F3** to save, or click on the **Save** button. Your information will then be added to the MultiLink List which will appear on the screen.

To exit the MultiLink screen, click on the **Close** button at the bottom of the screen.

Diagnosis List

This list contains the ICD-9 codes which represent a diagnosis of the illness or condition the patient is being treated for. This screen allows you to enter data on each diagnosis used in treating patients. In the real world, many providers and medical billers will purchase computerized ICD-9 code lists which can be automatically loaded into the computer each year. However, changes or updates to this list may need to be done manually.

To access the Diagnosis Codes List, click on the Diagnosis Codes List icon, or choose the **Lists** Menu option and choose **Diagnosis Codes**.

Exercise 5 – 8: Sue Pervisor gives you a list of diagnoses that were not entered into the system (Document 5). Look up the correct ICD-9 codes and enter the information for these diagnoses in the appropriate fields in the Diagnosis Codes List.

Code 1: Enter the diagnosis code, including any periods or additional classification numbers.

Description: Enter a description of the diagnosis. You are given more room than appears in the field. If you continue typing after hitting the field margin, the items first entered will scroll off the left side of the field, but will still be included in the complete description. However, it is important to be sure that all the pertinent data is included in the first part of the description line. When using the search feature, the first set of characters is the only ones to appear on the screen. Additionally, on many billing forms and reports, only the first part of the diagnosis appears. The remaining information will only appear on a walkout receipt that is printed in paragraph form.

Alternate Codes Sets: Code 2/3: If an alternate coding system is used by one or more of the insurance carriers, the alternate codes for the procedure listed can be entered here. The computer can then automatically choose the correct code to enter on the billing form. For example, if the Code Number 2 slot is used for state assigned codes and the insurance carrier listed in the Insurance Information file has a 2 in the Procedure Code Type Set, then any state assigned codes listed in this spot will automatically print on the billing form for that insurance carrier.

HIPAA Approved: Checking this box indicates that this code is HIPAA approved.

Inactive Code: Check this box if you need to deactivate a code, but not delete it. This may need to be done if an ICD-9 code has been deleted by the WHO, but all previous claims with this code have not yet been paid. If there are still open issues on the claims, the code needs to remain in the system. Having a code on an inactive status may prevent you from entering this code on new claims.

After entering diagnosis data, be sure to hit **F3** to save, or click on the **Save** button. Your information will then be added to the Diagnosis Code List which will appear on the screen.

To exit the Diagnosis Code screen, click on the **Close** button.

Summary

The Lists Menu choices allow you to enter information on the patient, providers, insurance carriers, addresses, procedure codes, and diagnoses. The information entered in these screens will be used to bill for the procedures performed by a provider, and to keep track of patient accounts. Data usually must be entered in these screens prior to being accessed in the Transaction Entry and Billing screens.

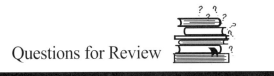

Questions for Review

Directions: Answer the following questions without looking back into the material just covered. Write your answers in the space provided.

1. What does EDI/EMC stand for? _____

   _____

2. In the Address List, what is a facility? _____

   _____

3. Name five advantages of EDI/EMC claims over paper claims.

   1. _____

      _____

   2. _____

      _____

   3. _____

      _____

   4. _____

      _____

   5. _____

      _____

4. What is the function of a clearinghouse? _____

   _____

   _____

   _____

5. What types of services would be considered patient only responsibility? _____

   _____

   _____

   _____

If you were unable to answer any of the questions, refer back to that section, and then fill in the answers.

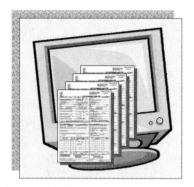

6

Patients/Guarantors and Cases List

After completion of this chapter you will be able to:

- Enter information on patients, guarantors and cases.
- Demonstrate use of the patient recall list.

Each patient and guarantor must be set up in this list in order to be accessed. The Patient List has two screens, containing all the data necessary to keep an accurate and complete patient file. Because the Patient Information and Case screens are so important, they will be handled in their own chapter. The remaining Lists Screens were covered in Chapter 5.

Case Based Files

MediSoft windows allows for patient files to be set up on a case basis. This means that you can track information regarding treatment on a specific incident. You can also keep track of two incidents and bill two separate insurance carriers.

For example, a patient may be seen on a regular basis for a diagnosis of hypertension. Then suddenly he has an injury at work. While his regular insurance carrier would be responsible for payment on all treatments relating to the hypertension, the employer's Workers' Compensation carrier would be responsible for payment on the services relating to the treatment of the work injury.

By setting up two separate case files for this patient, it is easy to keep the hypertension charges separate from the Workers' Compensation charges.

Depending on the circumstances of patient visits, a patient may have any number of files. Some practices choose to combine all patient visits under one file, unless they are billing a different insurance carrier.

While the case based file scenario allows for easy tracking of individual diagnoses and/or conditions, it can make it more confusing to track the number of times a patient visits the provider. Therefore, the provider should consider carefully when they want to establish a new case. For purposes of this text, all patients should be given a separate case file for each of the following situations:

1. Routine office visits and/or short term conditions/diseases (i.e., flu) should be lumped together under a single case file.
2. Chronic or long term conditions or diagnoses (those lasting longer than six months, such as pregnancy, diabetes, etc.) should each have their own separate case file.
3. Workers' Compensation Cases (including those which may possibly be related to Workers' Compensation) should be placed in a separate case file.
4. Accidents, especially those in which a third party may be at fault, should be placed in a separate case file.

Since the simulated work program encompasses such a short period of time, most patients will only have a single case file. However, care should be taken to remember the four situations listed above as some of them will be used and thus, separate case files will need to be set up for certain patients.

Patients/Guarantors and Cases List

This option allows you to enter data on a patient. It contains all the personal information needed on the patient, as well as additional information regarding specific encounters. Each patient, and each guarantor, whether they are a patient or not, must have their information set up in a file.

This menu option actually contains two separate lists which have their own data fields. The first is for entering information on patients and guarantors. The second is for entering more specific information regarding a case, the insurance carriers responsible for payment on the case, and other information.

Searching for a patient and deleting a patient are performed here in a similar manner to all other lists. (For further information, consult Chapter 5.) However, once a patient is chosen in the search field, a list of that patient's cases will appear in a second search screen to the right of the patient's name. This allows you to choose not only the patient you wish to work on, but also the specific case that you wish to work on.

If you wish to add a new patient, simply click on **New** or press **F8** while the cursor is in the patient portion of the screen. If you wish to add a new case to an existing patient, highlight the patient's name in the Case portion of the screen. The options at the bottom of the screen will now change to Edit Case, New Case, Delete Case, or Copy Case. This allows you to perform these functions without changing the patient information.

Patient/Guarantor List

There are two screens in the Patient/Guarantor List: the Name, Address screen and the Other Information screen.

Exercise 6 – 1: Take out the patient information sheets for the Dunnitt and Waite families (Documents 1 and 2). As you go through each of the following fields, enter the patient information as it pertains to the family. Each of the family members must be entered separately under their own patient chart number. Read through the description detailing each screen whether it pertains to this patient or not. It will help to familiarize you with the MediSoft System and its capabilities.

Not all screens or fields will be affected by the information given. For example, if the patient is not currently being treated, the condition screen may not be utilized. Also, there may not be any secondary or tertiary insurance coverage for family members.

Name, Address Screen
This screen is used for entering the patient's name and address, as well as other personal information about the patient.

Chart Number: Each patient must have their own individual patient chart number. Due to the configuration of the MediSoft system, each patient chart number must have eight digits (either letters or numbers). Each provider may choose their own system for setting up patient accounts, or you can allow MediSoft to assign chart numbers for each patient. For this course we will allow MediSoft to assign patient chart numbers. Be sure to write the patient chart number on the Patient Information Sheet.

Inactive: Check this box if you need to deactivate a patient, but not delete him/her. This may need to be done if a patient is no longer with the practice, but all the claims have not yet been paid. If there are still open issues on the claims of this patient, the patient needs to remain in the system. Having a patient on an inactive status may prevent you from entering new claims for this patient.

Last Name: Enter the last name of the patient. If the patient has a title designation at the end of their name (i.e., M.D., Jr., Sr., etc.), it should be entered directly after the last name.

First Name: Enter the patient's first name.

Middle Initial: Enter the patient's middle initial.

Street: Enter the street address of the patient.

City: Enter the city the patient lives in.

State: Enter the state in which the patient lives. This should coincide with the official postal two-letter state abbreviation.

Zip Code: Enter the patient's zip code. If the complete nine-digit zip code is known, enter the first five digits, a hyphen, and the remaining four digits.

Country: Enter the country in which the patient resides. This information is optional, but could be helpful for providers whose practices are near a country border.

E-mail: Enter the patient's e-mail address.

Home: Enter the patient's home phone number. Do not use parentheses or hyphens.

Work: If there is a work/office phone number for the patient, enter it here. Do not use parentheses or hyphens.

Cell: Enter the patient's personal cell phone number. Do not use parentheses or hyphens.

Fax: Enter the patient's fax phone number. Do not use parentheses or hyphens.

Other: Enter any other contact numbers for this patient (i.e., a pager number). Do not use parentheses or hyphens.

Birth Date: Enter the patient's birthdate in the MMDDYYYY format. If desired, you may click on the calendar to bring up and choose a date in the same manner you chose the date under File/Set Program Date.

Sex: Enter the sex of the patient: M for male, F for female. This should be the gender of the patient at the time services were rendered. If a patient enters the hospital for a sex change operation, it should be the gender of the patient as of the date they entered the hospital.

Birth Weight: Enter the birth weight of the patient, if known. This field is used for newborns or infants.

Units: Choose either grams or pounds to indicate the correct units for the weight entered in the previous field.

Social Security Number: Enter the patient's social security number. Do not enter hyphens.

Other Information Screen

This screen is used to indicate assigned provider, signature on file, and employment information on the patient or guarantor.

Type: Choose whether this person is a patient or a guarantor. A guarantor is someone who is financially responsible for a patient (i.e., a parent or guardian). This box is important when a dependent is being treated, but the insured is not. However, information for the insured is needed in order to properly process the insurance claims. This can often happen if the insured is a parent and the provider is a pediatrician treating the child.

What other instances can you think of where the insured may not be a patient, but the dependent may be?

_____
_____
_____
_____
_____
_____

Assigned Provider: Enter the code (from the provider listing) which corresponds to the doctor who is assigned to this patient. This information will automatically be transferred to the transaction entry and onto the billing forms. If another provider within the practice sees a patient (i.e., a patient is referred to a specialist within the group), this information will need to be changed so that the proper provider shows up on the patient's billing.

Patient ID #2: This box is an optional method for searching for a patient. Instead of searching for a patient by the chart number or the patient name, any key or combination of keys can be entered into this box to search for the patient. This can be a complete last name, nickname, company affiliation, or any other way which makes it easier to locate the record. This box is for internal use only and does not show up on insurance billing forms.

Patient Billing Code: This field allows you to sort patients into separate fields. The actual choice of groups was made in the Billing Codes field of the Lists Menu option. This field allows you to assign a patient to a specific group.

Patient Indicator: This field can be used as an additional sorting tool. You can create a five-digit code for any type of group.

For example: If you enter MEDCR and the Billing Code for this patient was Last Name A – M, sorting by both of these fields would allow you to locate all the Medicare patients whose last names began with A – M.

Flag Field: This field allows you to color code the patient file. You can color code patient records to alert you to various situations when those records are accessed in the program. Only one flag can be assigned to a patient record.

The patient's name will be shaded the chosen color in the Transaction Entry, Patient List, Quick Ledger, Deposit Entry, Apply Payment/Adjustments to Charges, List Only Claims That Match, Patient Recall, Quick Balance, Contact Log Entry, Eligibility Verification, Treatment Plan List, List Only Statements That Match, and Appointment Entry in Office Hours.

Healthcare ID: This is a code to help you identify the patient without revealing information about their identity (which may not be the case with a patient account number). This field has been created to help a practice maintain HIPAA compliance.

Signature on File: Place an X in the box if the patient's signature is on file authorizing release of medical information. If the patient's signature is not on file, the patient must sign the form prior to submitting it to the insurance carrier.

Signature Date: Enter the date on which the patient or guarantor signed the Release of Medical Information form. The signature on these forms is generally good for a period of one year unless stated otherwise on the form. A patient may revoke this signature by writing a letter to the practice stating that they no longer authorize the release of their information. This box is only activated if an X is placed in the Signature on File box.

Emergency Contact

The following fields allow you to enter emergency contact information for the patient.

Name: Enter the full name of the patient's emergency contact.

Home Phone: Enter the home phone number of the patient's emergency contact. Do not use parentheses or hyphens.

Cell Phone: Enter the cell phone number of the patient's emergency contact. Do not use parentheses or hyphens.

Default Employment Information for New Cases

Employer: Enter the employer address code. This item cross-references with information entered in the Addresses List. If this information has not yet been entered, you should enter it before you proceed.

You can press **F6** to search for an employer address code, or click on the magnifying glass to the right of this field. If the correct employer has not been entered, press **F8** and the Address List screen will appear. This will allow you to enter the new address before going on. (For instructions on completing the Address List screen, see Address List.)

Status: Most group insurance issued through an employer requires that the insured work full-time for the company. Additionally, dependents who work full-time may have duplicate coverage with their employer. Use this box to show the patient's work status as follows:

- Not Employed
- Full-time
- Part-time

- Retired
- Unknown

Work Phone: Indicate the work phone number for the patient. Do not use parentheses or hyphens.

Extension: Indicate the extension number at which the patient can be reached at work.

Location: This field can be used to indicate where in a company a person works. This can be an actual site (i.e., Tucson to indicate the patient works in the Tucson office), or a location within a site (i.e., warehouse, shop, or the name of a department).

Retirement Date: If the retirement date is known for this patient, indicate it here. This allows you to know when their insurance may terminate, or may change to a different plan. If a patient retires or terminates, but elects to continue coverage under COBRA rules, the biller should contact the employer to insure that the current monthly premium has been paid prior to the rendering of services.

Case Screens

Once you have entered the basic data on the patient, you need to enter the information regarding this case of treatment. If this person is the guarantor and not the patient, you will not need to access these screens.

The case screens will need to be completed in order to provide all the necessary information for completing the CMS-1500 form. Since some items on the form pertain to individual situations, having separate case screens allows you to keep each item separate.

While it may not be wise to create a new case file for each separate diagnosis of a patient certain situations will necessitate the creation of a separate case file. These can include:

1. **Standard Treatment.** All standard treatment for a patient should be kept under one case. Even if the specific incidents or reasons for treatment are not related, keeping items together can allow you to see the overall health of a patient and their treatment history.

2. **Chronic condition.** If a patient is receiving treatment for an ongoing (chronic) condition (i.e., diabetes), the provider may want this information entered into a separate case file. All treatments relating to this specific diagnosis can then be tracked. This may include regular checkups, or eventual blindness or amputation of a limb.

3. **Motor Vehicle Accident.** Often there is a third party liability, or other insurance (i.e., auto insurance) which may cover some or all of the costs related to a motor vehicle accident. Therefore, all treatment for injuries received in a specific motor vehicle accident should be kept separate from all other treatments.

4. **Workers' Compensation/Work Related Injury.** Any injury received on the job or that is related to work is often covered by the employer's Workers' Compensation policy. Treatment for these injuries should be separated from all other treatment so that the employer's insurance carrier can be accurately billed.

Personal Screen

This screen allows you to enter personal data regarding the patient and this specific case.

Case Number: The MediSoft program will automatically assign a case number. These numbers begin with one and continue consecutively.

Description: Enter a brief description of this case. This will help you to locate the proper case when using the search screen.

Guarantor: Enter the chart number for the guarantor for this treatment episode. In order for a guarantor chart number to work, the guarantor must have been previously entered as a patient or a guarantor in the Patient List. MediSoft will automatically enter the chart number of the patient. If this is incorrect, simply change it by typing in a new chart number or by searching for the correct chart number. You can easily access the search feature by clicking on the magnifying glass to the right of this field.

Print Patient Statement: If a patient or family should not receive a monthly statement, leave this box blank. If they should receive a statement, place an X in the box. This is an on/off field. Each time you click on the field, the X will appear or disappear. All CHS patients should receive statements.

Marital Status: Enter the marital status designation for the patient. These marital status designations correspond with those accepted on the CMS-1500 as follows:

- Divorced
- Legally Separated
- Married
- Single
- Unknown
- Widowed

Student Status: Many insurance plans cover a dependent until age 18 or 19, unless they are a full time student. Then coverage may be extended to age 23 or 24. This question will alert the insurance carrier that the patient is a student. Enter one of the following:

- Full Time Student
- Part Time Student
- Non-student
- If the student status is unknown, leave the field blank

Employment Section
Here you have an opportunity to change the employment information for the patient. If the patient has two jobs and this accident relates to a job other than that which they have their insurance through, this information could be important.

Data from the Patient List screen will automatically transfer into these fields. If the information is correct, simply tab past these fields. If it is incorrect, you can change it by clicking on the appropriate field and re-entering the data.

Employer: Enter the employer address code. This item cross-references with information entered in the Addresses List. If this information has not yet been entered, you should enter it before you proceed.

You can press **F6** to search for an employer address, or click on the magnifying glass to the right of this field. If the correct employer has not been entered, press **F8** and the Address List screen

will appear. This will allow you to enter the new address before going on.

Status: Most group insurance issued through an employer requires that the insured work full-time for the company. Additionally, dependents who work full-time may have duplicate coverage with their employer. Use this box to show the patient's work status as follows:

- Not Employed
- Full Time
- Part Time
- Retired
- Unknown

Retirement Date: If the retirement date is known for this patient, indicate it here. This allows you to know when their insurance may terminate, or may change to a different plan. If a patient retires or terminates, but elects to continue coverage under COBRA rules, the biller should contact the employer to insure that the current monthly premium has been paid prior to the rendering of services.

Location: This field can be used to indicate where in a company a person works. This can be an actual site (city), or a location within a site (i.e., warehouse, shop, or the name of a department).

Work Phone: Indicate the work phone number for the patient. Do not use parentheses or hyphens.

Extension: Indicate the extension number at which the patient can be reached at work.

Account Screen
Assigned Provider: Enter the code (from the Provider List) which corresponds to the doctor who is assigned to treat this specific case. This may or may not be the patient's normally assigned provider. For example, a specialist may be assigned to treat the patient's heart disease, but his regularly assigned physician continues to treat him for all other conditions.

If the provider has not been previously added to the Provider List, they will need to be added using the **F8** key.

Once the provider's code has been entered, the provider's name will appear to the right of the code.

Referring Provider: If this patient was referred by another provider, the referring physician and their UPIN need to be indicated on the billing forms (especially on Medicare claims). In order to use this field, the referring physician's information must have previously been entered in the Referring Providers List. If so, enter the physician's Referring Provider Code into this field.

If the referring provider has not been entered into the Referring Provider list, they will need to be added using the **F8** key.

Where does this information appear on a CMS-1500?

Supervising Provider: At times the work will be performed by one provider under the direction of another provider (i.e., a practitioner's assistant may provide services under the direction of the physician). In such a case the supervising provider's code will be entered here. This provider's information must have previously been entered into the provider listing.

Referral Source: Enter the Address Code for the person or entity that referred this patient. In order to have an Address Code, the person or entity must have been previously entered using the Address Lists screen. If they have not been entered, you can enter them by pressing the **F8** key.

This field is used to track how effective your advertising sources are. In order to gain the most effective report, entries must be identical. For example, if the patient was referred by Yellow Pages ad, all patients with the referral "Yellow Pages" will appear in a different listing from those referred by "Phone Listing." Common referral sources include a friend, telephone directories, other providers, pharmacists, radio, or other advertisements. It is possible to create a referral source for the above by placing the words "Yellow Pages" (or whatever else) in the name field of the Address List.

Attorney: If an attorney is associated with the care of this patient, enter the Address Code for that attorney in this field. Once again the attorney's information must have previously been entered into the Address Information data base.

Facility: If the patient was hospitalized or if services were provided at a facility other than the provider's office, enter the address code for the facility here. The address code must have been created in the Address List option. The entire name and address information for the facility will appear on the CMS-1500.

Where does the facility appear on the CMS-1500?

Case Billing Code: Often practices split their billing into several groups. This allows for continuous income during the month, as well as prevents the major backlog of work which can happen with billing all patients at once. Using this field, you can place patients into groups for billing purposes. Patients can be grouped together by last name (i.e., A – M is billed on the first of the month and N – Z is billed on the 15th of the month), insurance carrier or type of insurance, or any other form the practice wishes. The billing code must have been previously entered in the Billing Code List. Since we are using so few patients, we will bill them all at once. Therefore, you may leave this space blank.

Other Arrangements: There are four characters allowed in this field to indicate any special arrangements that have been made with the patient. These can involve items such as discounts, payment programs, or courtesy services (no billing). When new charges are entered for the patient on the Transaction Entry screen, this code is displayed at the bottom of the screen to remind you of the arrangements that have been made.

Treatment Authorized Through: Enter the date through which the insurance carrier has authorized treatments. Treatments received after this date may not be paid by the insurance carrier.

Visit Series

If treatment for the patient requires a series of visits, pre-authorization may be needed to determine the number of treatments the insurance carrier will cover (i.e., up to 12 massage therapy visits may be covered for a patient with a back injury). The following fields are for entering information on a series of visits.

Authorization Number: The pre-authorization number provided by the carrier should be entered in this field. This number usually identifies the person authorizing the treatments.

Authorized Number of Visits: Enter the number of visits which have been authorized.

ID: This field allows for several visit series to be monitored at once. Enter a letter A – Z to indicate the series. Most often an A is entered. The computer will automatically count the number of visits, up to the pre-authorized limit number, then switch to the next letter in the series. Different series IDs may be used for subsequent series of the same problem, or for different problems which require a series of treatments.

Last Visit Date: MediSoft automatically enters the date of the last visit entered in the Transaction Entry screen. If this date needs to be modified, enter the corrected information.

Last Visit Number: Each time a visit is entered in the Transaction Entry screen, this number is increased by one until it reaches the limit entered in the Authorized Number of Visits field. This number is normally not edited by the medical biller.

Diagnosis Screen
This screen is for entering diagnoses and diagnosis codes associated with this patient's treatment.

Default Diagnosis 1, 2, 3, 4: These fields are for entering the patient's diagnoses. Since MediSoft handles charges on a case basis, often the diagnoses for all treatments within a case will be the same.

Since many cases will relate to the same diagnoses, entering the diagnoses in this field will save time.

Enter the diagnosis codes associated with this patient. If no code is entered, the diagnosis entered during the first transaction entry will automatically become the default code and will be entered in the first space.

Allergies and Notes: Enter any allergies or special notes associated with this patient. This information will appear at the bottom of the Transaction Entry screen, but it will not print anywhere. While entering the information for the Dunnitt and Waite

families, be sure to check if any data should be entered here.

EDI/EMC Notes
This window allows the entry of additional data that is included with electronic claims when they are submitted. If the provider is an anesthesiologist, enter the symbol @ (shift 2). The first 17 characters entered after this symbol will print on the claim form. This allows entry of documentation such as Time: 12:00-14:50 which is needed for claim processing.

If the practice type in the Practice Information screen was listed as Chiropractic, an additional field will be added for **Level of Subluxation**. The subluxation level is indicated by where the subluxation occurs (C1, T2, L3, etc.). This information is often required by insurance carriers when a patient is treated by a chiropractor.

Using a medical dictionary and/or other resource materials, answer the following questions.

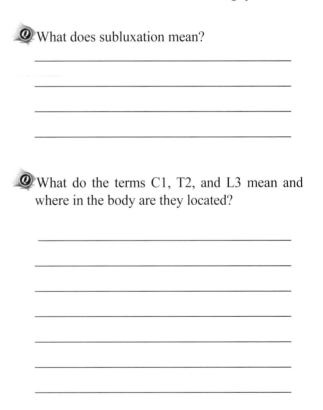

What does subluxation mean?

_____

_____

_____

_____

What do the terms C1, T2, and L3 mean and where in the body are they located?

_____

_____

_____

_____

_____

_____

_____

Condition Screen
The Condition Screen contains information that pertains to this specific episode of treatment. This information is used to properly complete the CMS-1500 form. At this time you will not enter condition

information for the Dunnitt and Waite families. This data will be completed when treatment commences.

While reading through this section, compare these fields with the boxes to be completed on the CMS-1500. Next to each item, indicate the CMS-1500 box number. If there is no corresponding box number on the CMS-1500, enter NONE on the line given.

Injury/Illness/LMP Date: Enter the date on which the illness or injury occurred. If this condition is related to a pregnancy, enter the date of the patient's last menstrual period (LMP). If the onset of the illness was gradual, enter a G and the word gradual will appear on the form. Entering N will print N/A in this field.

Where does this information appear on a CMS-1500?

_____

Illness Indicator: Enter an I to indicate if the date given in the previous box pertains to an illness or injury. Enter an L to indicate the date is the last menstrual period, or you may click on the ↓ to the right of the field and a list of these choices will appear.

First Consultation Date: Enter the date on which the provider first began treating this patient for this condition.

Date Similar Symptoms: If the patient has had similar symptoms in the past that are not related to this specific episode of treatment (i.e., tonsillitis patient had a previous tonsillitis experience two years ago), enter the date those symptoms occurred.

Where does this information appear on a CMS-1500?

_____

Same/Similar Symptoms: Enter an X in this box for Yes, similar symptoms occurred on the date entered. Leave the box blank if no similar symptoms have appeared.

Employment Related: Enter an X in this box if this condition is related to the patient's employment.

This is most often used when a person is injured on the job, but the condition could also be a chronic condition which is due to their job. For example, if a person repeatedly uses their fingers to type, they may suddenly be seized with a sharp pain in their wrist while doing weekend gardening. The doctor may diagnose the condition as carpal tunnel syndrome. While the initial reason for visiting the doctor was pain from gardening, the underlying cause of the condition is likely the constant typing done while at work.

If the condition is work related, Workers' Compensation laws may cover payment on this claim. An empty box indicates the claim is not work-related.

Where does this information appear on a CMS-1500?

_____

Emergency: Enter an X in this box if these procedures were provided on an emergency basis. Leave the box blank if they were not.

Where does this information appear on a CMS-1500?

_____

Accident Information

If these services were related to an accident, information regarding the accident can be entered in this section.

Related To: Enter a Y if this claim is related to an accident, an A if it is related to an auto accident, and an N if it is not related to an accident. Or you can click on the ↓ to the right of the field for a list of these choices. It is important to determine the accident status of each and every claim since additional benefits may be available for accidents. Additionally, if the accident involved another party (i.e., an auto accident or negligence on the part of another person or company) third party liability laws might cover payment on this claim.

If an A is placed in this box, where will this information appear on a CMS-1500?

_____

Look at Document 16 in the back of this book. Does the Ball Insurance Carriers contract have an accident benefit? If so, what does it say?

_____

_____

_____

_____

_____

How can this benefit affect payment on an accident claim?

_____

_____

_____

_____

State: List the two-digit postal code for the state in which the accident occurred if the accident is auto related. This helps to determine the laws and rules which govern coverage of a two-party accident, since many states have different laws and rules.

Where does this information appear on a CMS-1500?

_____

Nature of Accident: If this claim pertains to an accident, choose one of the following codes:
- Injured at Home
- Injured at School
- Injured during recreation
- Motorcycle Injury
- Work Injury/Non-collision
- Work Injury/Self-Employed
- Some states require this code when submitting claims electronically

Dates Unable to Work: Enter the beginning and ending dates of the time the patient is unable to work.

Where does this information appear on a CMS-1500?

_____

Total Disability: Enter the beginning and ending dates of the time the patient is to be considered totally disabled.

Partial Disability: Enter the beginning and ending dates of the time the patient is to be considered partially disabled.

Hospitalization: Enter admit and discharge dates for a hospitalized patient.

Where does this information appear on a CMS-1500?

_____

Last X-ray Date: Some insurance carriers require the date of the last x-ray. This is usually for chiropractic patients who are eligible for Medicare. If needed, enter the date of the last x-ray.

Death/Status: D. A. Karnofsky, a 20th-century physician developed a scale to indicate a patient's physical state, performance, and prognosis. The scale ranges from 100; perfectly well, to 0; dead. Some carriers require the reporting of the patient's condition on a similar scale. The code to be entered in this box is based upon the scale Karnofsky developed. Appropriate codes are (from worst to best) as follows:
- Dead (Medicare Assigned claims only)
- Moribund (dying)
- Very sick
- Severely disabled
- Disabled
- Requires considerable assistance
- Requires occasional assistance
- Cares for self
- Normal activity with effort
- Able to carry on normal activity
- Normal

Return to Work Indicator: Enter an L if the patient is allowed to return to work with limited activity. Enter an N if the patient is allowed to resume normal work activity. Enter a C if the return to work is conditional. Or you may click on the ↓ to the right of the field to get a list of these choices.

Percent of Disability: Once a patient's condition is stabilized and no additional progress is expected to be made, the physician will list the patient as permanently disabled. This percentage indicator reflects the amount of disability which the patient will likely have for the remainder of their life. This can range from 1 – 2% for a permanently disabled toe to 100% for a totally disabled patient.

Pregnant: Place an X in this box if the patient is pregnant.

Estimated Date of Birth: Enter the estimated date of birth for this pregnancy.

Date Assumed Care:/Date Relinquished Care: These fields are provided for situations in which two different providers share the care of one episode of treatment. For example, if one provider is responsible for the pre-partum care and delivery, and a different provider is responsible for the post-partum delivery. These fields allow you to indicate the dates a specific provider assumed and relinquished care for the patient.

Miscellaneous Screen

This screen is used for additional information relating to this claim or this case of treatment.

Outside Lab Work: Enter an X in this box if an outside lab billed for services related to this claim.

Where does this information appear on a CMS-1500?

_____

Lab Charges: Enter the amount of the outside lab charges in this box.

Where does this information appear on a CMS-1500?

_____

Local Use A: This box completes any information needed for item 10d on the CMS-1500. Currently this box is used by Medicare to indicate secondary payors or items needed to process Medicare claims.

If this item is required by your Medicare carrier, they will specify the code or item they want in this field.

Local Use B: This box completes any information needed for item 19 on the CMS-1500. This box is used by states and localities to indicate information they need in claim processing.

Indicator: If further delineation is needed in setting up billing cycles, this field may be used with the Billing Code field to create an unlimited array of billing groups.

Referral Date: Enter the date of referral.

Prescription Date: Enter the date a prescription was given.

Prior Authorization #: If pre-authorization is required for certain procedures or treatments, a pre-authorization number will be supplied by the carrier in regards to these services. If a pre-authorization number has been obtained for any of the services on this claim, enter the number in this box. Pre-authorization is also sometimes called pre-certification.

Where does this information appear on a CMS-1500?

_____

Look at Document 17 in the back of this book. What procedures require pre-authorization on the Rover Insurers contract?

_____

_____

_____

_____

_____

_____

Extra 1/2/3/4: These fields are to allow extra information needed in processing this claim. Enter any additional information pertaining to the patient. Since MediSoft has the ability to sort by this field, a provider may wish to categorize his patients and enter certain categories here. This will allow the provider to determine, for example, how many AIDS patients or diabetes patients he is treating.

Outside Primary Care Provider: This field allows information to be entered regarding a primary care provider for the patient who is not a member of this practice. This field is most often used when the provider is a specialist and was referred by an outside primary care physician. This space is for the address code. In order to enter this provider, their information must have previously been entered in the Address List screen.

Date Last Seen: Enter the date this patient was last seen by the outside primary care provider.

Policy 1 Screen
Homebound: Check this box if the patient is homebound.

Policy 1
This screen allows you to enter information on the primary insurance coverage for this patient.

Insurance 1: Enter the code number for the insurance company. The code number comes from the Insurance Carriers List. If you are unsure of the insurance carrier number, press **F6** or click on the magnifying glass and search for it. If the insurance carrier has not been entered, press **F8** to add the insurance carrier.

Policy Holder 1: Enter the chart number of the primary insured. This may be the patient (self), or a spouse or parent of the patient. Enter the correct patient chart number, or press **F6** (or click on the magnifying glass) to search for it.

Relationship to Insured: Enter the relationship of the patient to the insured according to the code choices below:
- Self
- Spouse
- Child
- Other

NOTE: In this case, the term "Child" includes natural children, adopted children, and step-children. If the relationship is "Other," it would be appropriate to enter the relationship information in the Allergies/Notes section in the condition screen.

Policy Number: Enter the patient's policy number. This is the number issued by the insurance carrier to help them keep track of the plan the insured is covered under. This is the ID# under the insurance carrier name located on the Patient Information Sheet.

Group Number: Enter the patient's group number as issued by the insurance carrier. Not all insurance carriers will issue both a policy number and a group number. Some will issue only one or the other, some will issue a group name rather than a group number.

Claim Number: This field is required for some electronic claims. It is used on property/casualty/ auto claims. This number is assigned by the property and casualty payer.

Policy Dates Start/End: Enter the beginning and ending dates of the policy. If the policy is still current, no date need be entered in the Stop field. This information is important when submitting claims to help insure that the patient is actually covered at the time services are rendered. When a biller is making an appointment for the patient for a date in the future, this box should be checked to insure that the patient still has insurance coverage on that date.

Assignment of Benefits/Accept Assignment: Does the provider accept Medicare Assignment on this patient? Place an X in the box for yes. Leave the box blank for no.

Capitated Plan: Is this patient a member of a capitated plan? If so, the provider receives a monthly payment which covers most services rendered to this patient. If an X is entered in this box, the insurance coverage percent should indicate that the plan pays 100% of the charges. It is important for the biller to be aware of those charges that are not covered by the capitation amount and which should be billed on a fee-for-service basis.

These items should be billed separately, under a separate case file. Normally services rendered which fall under the capitation plan will not require a bill to be generated; however, a record of procedures performed should be kept to assist the provider in understanding the cost of services rendered and in reporting to the carrier.

Deductible Met: Check this box if the patient has previously met their deductible. This field will help to determine the proper amount for the patient's portion of the visit.

Annual Deductible: Enter the amount of the patient's annual deductible. This field will also help to determine the proper amount for the patient's portion of the visit.

Copayment Amount: If the patient is part of a managed care plan which requires a copayment to be collected from the patient at the time of the visit, the copayment amount should be entered in this field. When entering charges in the Transaction Entry screen, this amount will appear at the bottom of the screen to remind you to collect these fees from the patient at the time of the visit.

Insurance Coverage Percents by Service Classification: Enter the standard coinsurance percentage which the insurance carrier pays. This information is used to calculate the estimated patient responsibility amount (i.e., on an 80/20 plan the insurance covers 80% of the charge and the patient is responsible for the other 20%). This amount will show up at the bottom of the Transaction Entry screen when charges are entered. Some providers prefer to have this amount collected from the patient at the time services are rendered, while others wait until the insurance carrier has paid their portion and then bill the patient for any amounts not covered. However, MediSoft does not calculate any remaining deductible amount.

Policy 2 and Policy 3 Screens
The information in these screens is entered the same as for the Policy 1 screen above. The Policy 2 screen is for the secondary payor and the Policy 3 screen is for the tertiary payor. If there is no secondary or tertiary payor, these screens should be left blank.

Medicaid and TRICARE Screen
This screen is for entering information on Medicaid and TRICARE patients.

EPSDT: The Early and Periodic Screening, Diagnosis, and Treatment program is intended to provide free or low cost care to Medicaid infants. The attempt is to provide basic medical services to infants to prevent a minor problem from becoming a major or lifelong one. Check this box if the service provided on this line is related to the EPSDT program.

Where does this information appear on a CMS-1500?

_____

Family Planning: If these services are related to Family planning, check this box.

Where does this information appear on a CMS-1500?

_____

Resubmission #/Original Reference: If Medicaid rejects a claim or sends it back for further information, often approval is required before resubmitting the claim. The Medicaid office will provide a resubmission number and an original reference number for the claim. These numbers should be entered in the appropriate boxes.

Where does this information appear on a CMS-1500?

_____

Service Authorization Exception Code: This code is required on some Medicaid claims. If you did not receive a service authorization code before seeing the patient, select one of the following codes:
1 Immediate/Urgent Care
2 Services Rendered in a Retroactive Period
3 Emergency Care
4 Client as Temporary Medicaid
5 Request from County for Second Opinion to Recipient can Work
6 Request for Override Pending
7 Special Handling

TRICARE

This section is used for treating TRICARE patients at a non-military facility or provider's location. Much of the information will be available on the patient's TRICARE card, or from the patient themselves.

Non-availability Indicator: Click on the ↓ to the right of this field to get a list of the choices indicated and enter one of the following indicators to show the patient's status:

- **YA** Non-availability statement obtained. This indicates that there is no available military facility convenient to the patient and he/she therefore has permission to seek treatment at a non-military facility.
- **NA** Non-availability statement not needed.
- **Z** Other carrier paid at least 75% of this claim.

Or you may click on the ↓ to the right of this field to get a list of the choices indicated.

Branch of Service: Enter the appropriate branch of the military which the patient is connected with. Choices include:

- Air Force
- Army
- Champ VA (Veterans)
- Coast Guard
- Marines
- Navy
- Public Health Service
- NOAA

Sponsor Status: Enter one of the following to indicate the patient's military status.

- 100% Disabled
- Academy Student/Navy OCS
- Active
- Civilian
- Deceased
- Foreign Military
- Former Member
- Medal of Honor
- National Guard
- Other
- Permanently Disabled
- Recalled to Active Duty
- Reserves
- Retired

- Temporarily Disabled
- Unknown

Special Program Indicator: If applicable, a code can be entered to indicate a special program under which the patient is covered. Applicable codes are:

- 03   Special Federal Funding
- 05   Disability
- 06   PPV/Medicare 100% Payment
- 07   Induced Abortion – Danger to Women's life
- 08   Induced Abortion – Victim of Rape/Incest
- 09   Second Opinion/Surgery
- 30   Medicare demo proj. for lung surgery study
- A   Patient is sponsor
- B   Patient is spouse
- C1   Patient is child 1
- C2   Patient is child 2
- C3   Patient is child 3
- C4   Patient is child 4
- C5   Patient is child 5
- C6   Patient is child 6
- C7   Patient is child 7
- C8   Patient is child 8
- C9   Patient is child 9
- D   Patient is widow of sponsor
- 70   Local use*
- 71   Local use*
- 72   Local use*
- 73   Local use*
- 74   Local use*
- 75   Local use*
- 76   Local use*
- 77   Local use*
- 78   Local use*
- 79   Local use*
- 80   Local use*

* These codes are to be assigned by your local carrier.

Sponsor Grade: Enter the appropriate pay grade for the patient:

- W1 – W4   Warrant Officer
- E1 – E9   Enlisted
- 01 – 11   Officer
- VA   CHAMPVA
- 19   Academy Student/Navy OCS
- 41 – 58   GS1 – GS10

- G1   G1
- S1   S1
- 90   Unknown
- 99   Other

Effective Dates Start/End: Enter the date TRICARE coverage became effective as shown on the patient's TRICARE card and the date on which TRICARE coverage did or will terminate for this patient.

After entering the patient and case data, be sure to hit **F3** to save, or click on the **Save** button. Your information will then be added to the Patient/Guarantor List which will appear on the screen.

To exit the Patient/Guarantor screen, click on the **Close** button at the bottom of the screen.

Deleting a Patient

Before deleting a patient, you must be sure they have no current transactions, no outstanding balances, and no dependents.

If there are any current transactions, you will need to wait until after the next month-end processing. The month-end processing will move these transactions into history.

If there is an outstanding balance, it will need to be adjusted off. Determine if there is an outstanding balance by printing a patient ledger. If there is an outstanding balance, you can enter an adjustment in the transaction entry screen to bring the balance to zero.

The above procedure should be done for each dependent and head of household before they are deleted. Then delete the dependents prior to deleting the head of household.

To delete a patient, go into the Patient List screen. You will automatically be entered into the search screen. Click on the patient or case you wish to delete and press **Delete Patient**. You will be asked to confirm that you want to delete this information. Click on either **Yes** or **No**.

It is possible to delete a specific case without deleting the information for the entire patient. To do this, simply click on the patient, then click on the specific case you wish to delete prior to hitting the delete key.

If the patient still has transactions or outstanding balances, you may choose to place them on inactive status rather than deleting them.

By clicking on the inactive button in the Patient Information screen, no new claims may be entered for this patient.

Printing a Patient Ledger

It is possible to print a patient ledger for a single patient while you are in the Patient Lists option, highlight the patient and case you wish to print a ledger for and press **F7**, or click on the **F7** Ledger symbol at the bottom of the screen.

You can also print patient ledgers through the Reports Menu option.

Patient Recall List

The Patient Recall List allows a practice to have a list of those patients who should be called for an additional appointment. This is most often used when the patient has a condition which necessitates a number of visits or continuous monitoring. For example, a patient with cancer in remission may need a visit and tests every six months to ensure that the cancer has not returned.

This list has the ability to be sorted by chart number, provider, or date. This allows the practice to print out a list of all the patients who should be recalled on a specific date, or patients who need to be scheduled for a visit with a specific provider.

To enter information on a patient who needs to be recalled, click on the Patient Recall Entry icon at the top of the screen or choose Patient Recall in the Lists menu and fill in the following fields:

Recall Date: Enter the date on which the patient should be recalled for a follow-up appointment.

Provider: Enter the code number for the provider the patient is to see. The provider must have been previously entered in the Provider List.

Chart: Enter the chart number of the patient. The patient must have previously been entered in the Patients/ Guarantors List.

Name: If you entered a chart number in the above field, the name should automatically appear in this field. This allows you to have the name handy so that you can refer to the patient by name when you make the recall, rather than by chart number.

Phone: The phone number which was entered for the patient in the Patients/Guarantors list should appear here.

Extension: If the patient's extension number does not automatically appear, enter it here.

Procedure: Indicate the procedure code for the service which the patient is being recalled for. This is most often an office visit. This allows you to know how long of an appointment the patient will need.

Message: Indicate any message for the patient. This may be an explanation of why they are to follow-up with the provider (i.e., to run tests to ensure that cancer has not returned).

Recall Status: These buttons allow you to keep track of the recall process. Upon first entering the data for a recall, the **Call** button will be highlighted. If you have called once and did not receive an answer, you would click on the **Call Again** button to indicate that at least one call was previously made to the patient. The **Appointment Set** button indicates that the call was successful and an appointment has been set for this patient. The **No Appointment** button indicates that you were successful in reaching the patient and spoke with them, however, the patient refused to set up an appointment at that time.

Summary

The Patients/Guarantors screens contain personal information on the patient. Case screens include information about the insurance policies covering the patient, the condition for which they are being treated, and their account. Most screens will only need to be updated when information changes, however the Condition screen should be checked each time a patient visits the doctor and before billing on a CMS-1500 form.

MediSoft also has a Recall List in the List Menu which allows you to keep track of all patients who need to be contacted regarding a follow-up appointment.

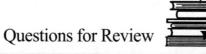

Questions for Review

Directions: Answer the following questions without looking back into the material just covered. Write your answers in the space provided.

1. List the four categories used for setting up case files?

    1. _____

        _____

    2. _____

        _____

    3. _____

        _____

    4. _____

        _____

2. What is the purpose of having case based files? _____

    _____

    _____

3. What is the purpose of the Patient Recall List? _____

    _____

4. Before deleting a patient you must be sure they have no _____

    _____ or _____

5. What does the EDI/EMC notes window allow? _____

    _____

    _____

If you were unable to answer any of the questions, refer back to that section, and then fill in the answers.

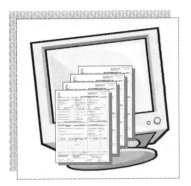

7

Activities Menu Options

The Activities menu option allows you to Enter Transactions, perform Claims Management, and use the Appointment Book. Most activities involving the patient occur in the Enter Transactions screen. The Appointment Entry screen in the Appointment Book is used to enter appointments. Since the Appointment Book option opens an entirely new computer program called the MediSoft Office Hours program, it will be discussed in its own chapter.

Transaction Entry

All charges, adjustments, payments, copayments, credits, lab charges, and general comments are entered into the patient's record through the Transaction Entry screen.

Go back to the information entered in the Procedure/Payment/Adjustment Code List to see the types of entries that are available using this screen. Each of the options entered in the procedure information screen will be added to a patient chart through the Enter Transactions screen. This screen is the one most often used by the medical biller during the course of normal operations.

Exercise 7 – 1: Sue Pervisor steps up to your desk with the following request. "Ben Waite just received a problem focused, straightforward exam ($55) performed by Dr. Phil Goode. He was hit in the head by a golf ball and has a head contusion. His mother will be down in a minute. She's in a hurry, but she wants to make a payment. Please enter this charge into the system so the bill will be ready."

As you read through the following information, enter this charge into the system. Use the date (January 2, 20XX) in the YYMMDD order as the document number.

Also remember that information concerning the patient's condition may need to be added in the Patient Information record, and Condition Screen.

You may need to look up the procedures and diagnoses in the CPT® and ICD-9 books. These codes will be entered during the entry of this patient's charges if they were not previously entered in the Procedure/ Payment/Adjustments List and Diagnosis List screens.

Chart: Enter the patient's chart number. If you do not know the patient's full chart number, this box has an automatic search feature. Simply begin entering the chart number and the first matching entry will pop up on the screen. This feature will bring up every chart number which matches the characteristics of the data you entered. If there is more than one choice, they will be listed in a search screen. If there is only one match to your entry, the chart number for that person will appear on the screen. If you do not know the chart number you may search for the patient by pressing **F6** or clicking on the magnifying glass icon.

Once a patient chart number has been chosen, the patient's name and birth date will appear to the right of the chart number. This can help you to insure that you have chosen the correct patient.

Case: Enter the number for the case of treatment to which these entries will be associated. It is important to match the transaction entries with the correct case scenario in order to correctly bill and apply transactions and payments. If only one case has been entered for this patient, it will appear in this field and the diagnosis will appear to the right of the field.

Briefcase Icon: To the right of the case field is a briefcase icon. This icon allows you to search for a case by a transaction date, procedure code, or amount. This can be very helpful when an insurance carrier has made a payment on a claim. The Explanation of Benefits (EOB) often will not list the diagnosis. Therefore, by matching either the transaction date, procedure code, or amount, you can find the correct case file. This can be very important since you must be in the proper case file for payments to be properly posted to their charges.

Clicking on the briefcase icon will bring up an additional search screen. Here you have the option to enter a date in the **Date From** field, a procedure code in the **Code** field, or an amount in the **Amount** field. If you choose, you may enter information in more than one field. Doing so will further limit the selections. For example, if you have an EOB which lists an office visit on a specific date, along with several other procedures, entering both a date and a procedure will further help the MediSoft program to choose the correct case which the payment applies to.

In the Charge and Payment/Adjustment/ Comment Screens, you are able to create, edit, and delete transactions. To create a new entry, click **New** and a new transaction field set will be added with the current date. You may change the date by typing in a different date. To delete an entry, click **Delete**. To edit an entry, click on the field you wish to edit and enter the new information.

Charge Entry Screen

Dates: MediSoft automatically enters the current date. If this date is not correct, enter the correct date of the charge (service), in the MMDDYY format. If there is a from and through date associated with the service, enter both dates. If you enter a date, that date will continue to be automatically entered as long as you are in the Enter New Transactions screen. This allows you to enter all charges from a certain day without reentering the date each time. If only one date is entered, MediSoft will print the same date in both date spaces of the CMS-1500.

Procedure: Enter the appropriate procedure code. This is usually a CPT® or HCPCS code for a medical procedure. If you do not know the code, it can be looked up by pressing **F6** or by clicking on the magnifying glass to the right of the field and searching for the information. If the information has not been entered in the Procedure Code List screen, you may access this screen by pressing **F8**. Once the information has been entered, press **F3** to save (or click on the **Save** button) and you will be returned to the Transaction Entry screen.

Units: Enter the number of days, times, or units this service was provided. The default setting is 1. If a number other than 1 is entered and you placed an X in the Multiply Units Times Amount box in the Program Options (File/Program Options), MediSoft will automatically multiply the number of units by the amount and enter the result in the Amount column.

Where on the CMS-1500 will the number of units show up?

_____

Amount: If the Procedure code listed was a CPT® code, MediSoft will automatically enter the amount for the procedure which was entered into the Procedure Code List. If this default amount is incorrect or is unavailable, type in the new amount.

Total: The total amount of the transactions will appear here. If the system is not set up to automatically multiply the units by the amount, you may need to enter the total amount in this field.

Diag 1/2/3/4: Enter the diagnosis code(s) for this episode of treatment. This is especially important when billing for charges as insurance carriers will not pay claims where no diagnosis is indicated. MediSoft allows you to enter up to four diagnosis codes. If there are more diagnosis codes, the transaction entries should be split. Enter all transactions that correspond to one, two, three, or four diagnoses on one screen, save the data, and then enter the additional procedures for any remaining diagnoses on a separate entry.

Diagnosis Boxes 1, 2, 3, 4: Place a ☑ in the box for each diagnosis which relates to this procedure. The applicable diagnoses were entered in the upper-right of the screen.

Provider: Enter the code for the physician who provided this service to the patient. The default setting is the Assigned Provider which was entered in the Patient Information screen.

POS (Place of Service): This code indicates the location where the procedure was performed. For a complete listing, see the CMS-1500 instructions or the back of many CMS-1500 forms. If you listed a default location code in the Procedure List screen, this code will automatically appear in this space. If it is incorrect, change it by typing in the new location code.

TOS (Type of Service): Enter the type of service for this charge/procedure. This field is often left blank.

Allowed: This field lists the Medicare allowed amount for this procedure.

MultiLink: If you want to enter a MultiLink code, click on the MultiLink button. This will bring up a new screen that allows you to enter the MultiLink code.

M1/M2/M3 (Modifiers): Enter the modifiers, if any, associated with this procedure.

Note: If there are any notes to be associated with this claim, enter them here.

The following fields are not present in the 2004 MediSoft version but may appear in earlier versions:

Payments/Adjustments/Comments Entry Screen
The Payments/Adjustments/Comments Entry screen allows you to enter payments, adjustments, and comments which have been made on a patient's account.

Exercise 7 – 2: Ova Waite steps up to the window with her son and states, "I've just seen the doctor and I want to make a payment on the bill."
She takes out her checkbook and hands you check #1234, bank # 11-111, in the amount of $30. Enter this payment in the Transaction Entry screen.

Date: MediSoft automatically enters the current date. If this date is not correct, enter the correct date of the payment in the MMDDYY format.

Pay/Adj Code: Enter the appropriate code for the type of payment or adjustment. These codes should previously have been entered using the Procedures/Payments/ Adjustments List screen. The Pay/Adj Code alerts MediSoft as to whether this is a payment or an adjustment.

Who Paid: Enter the name of the person who made this payment. Clicking on the ↓ to the right of this field will bring up several options. If you are unable to find the correct person, it means they have not been entered in the Patient/Guarantor List or Insurance List. They will need to be entered before they can be placed in this field.

Description: If the procedure was a payment by check, enter the check number, followed by the bank number (i.e., ck #1099, 16-999). If the procedure was an adjustment, enter the reason for the adjustment. For example, if you incorrectly coded a claim, enter incorrect coding and include the incorrect code along with the new, corrected code. This information is necessary when providers' accounts are audited.

Provider: Enter the code for the physician who provided this service to the patient. The default setting is the Assigned Provider which was entered into the Patient Information screen.

Amount: Enter the amount of the payment. MediSoft automatically recognizes that this is a payment and subtracts all payments from charges. Therefore, a minus (-) sign in front of the amount is not necessary. Since Adjustments can be either a credit (added to the account) or a debit (subtracted from the account), enter a minus sign in front of the amount for debit adjustments.

Check Number: Enter the check number here.

Unapplied: If the amount of the check is greater than the amount owed, there will be an unapplied amount. The program will automatically calculate this amount.

Apply: The Apply button applies payment to the charges. This does not appear in all versions of MediSoft.

Previous Versions of MediSoft

In previous versions of MediSoft, the Payment and Adjustment entries had two separate screens. The information that goes in each field is still the same. The following are fields which do not appear in the 2004 version of MediSoft but may appear in earlier versions:

Document: This is one of the most important numbers in the Transaction Entry screen. This number is used to tie all charges and payments together. Therefore it is vitally important that this number be the same for all entries which relate to each other. For example, if a patient is seen by the doctor on 10/1/XX and incurs charges of $500, the document number for the charges, the insurance payment, the patient payment, and any write-off should all carry the same document number. This allows you to see how much is outstanding on each bill, rather than just on the account as a whole.

A document number may be an invoice number, a date, a charge number, or any other number the practice chooses. MediSoft automatically enters the current date in the YYMMDD format. For purposes of this book, we will use the date of services as the document number.

Apply Payments to Charges: This field allows you to apply the payment to the correct charge. For example, a patient may be treated for a fractured leg and their insurance covers procedures, but does not cover durable medical equipment (i.e., crutches). They may want to make a payment on the crutches, but wants to wait until the insurance carrier has paid before making a payment on the visit.

When each entry has been completed you are ready to end the transaction. The icons on the right of the transaction screen allow you to perform the following functions (the keystrokes in parentheses can also be used to complete the function.):

1. Saves this transaction and then opens a new transaction (Shift **F3**). This function is used when you have additional transactions to enter.
2. Saves this transaction and closes the new transaction panel (**F3**). This function is used when you are finished entering transactions for this patient.
3. Abandon any changes or entries without saving.
4. Enter Transaction Documentation. This is a screen in which you are able to type notes regarding this transaction. These notes are used to substantiate services, or to reflect information which should be known regarding these procedures. This screen can be especially important when submitting electronic claims, since this is the only additional documentation which can be sent to substantiate the medical necessity of services. You are allowed up to 255 characters. There are eight types of Transaction Documentation:
   1. Operative Note: A note to substantiate the cause for operative procedures.
   2. Other: Miscellaneous notes which are important for correct processing of this claim.
   3. Oxygen Prescription: A prescription for oxygen therapy or equipment.
   4. PEN Certification: Prescription for parenteral therapy.
   5. Physical Therapy Certification: Notes to substantiate the need for physical therapy services.
   6. Prosthetics/Orthotics Certification: A prescription for prosthetic or orthotic

equipment, or notes to substantiate the need for such services.

7. Statement Note: A note which appears on the patient statement to explain additional charges, adjustments, etc.

8. Transaction Note: A note which is generated for internal use only and will not appear on the claim forms submitted to the carrier.

Transaction Entry Screen Display

In the upper-right-hand corner is a pair of boxes that summarizes some of the information for this and previous transactions to assist in properly billing the patient. It contains information about the patient and their account.

Last Visit Date and Visit # of #: If the insurance carrier authorized a series of visits for this patient (i.e., ten chiropractic visits for a back injury), these fields will display the date of the last visit and the number of visits which have been completed. It will also show the number of visits which were authorized. This allows you to warn the patient if they are nearing the end of the number of visits authorized.

Last Payment Date and Last Payment Amount: These fields display the date and amount of the last payment made on this patient. This information is taken from all previous entries in the transaction screen.

Estimated Responsibility Amounts (Policy 1, 2, 3): MediSoft will automatically calculate the estimated insurance payment by each payor, based upon the information entered in the Insurance List. For example, if the patient had only one insurance carrier and they covered all procedures at 80%, then 80% of the charges entered would be shown in this space.

Guarantor: This field shows the estimated amount of the guarantor's responsibility (i.e., the remaining 20% which the insurance does not cover). Any deductible not paid, allowed amounts, or other items which may affect payment are not calculated into either the Insurance or Patient Share fields.

Adjustments: This field shows any adjustments that have been entered on this account.

Policy Copay: The amount of copayment is shown here. This is the amount that should be collected from the patient at the time services are rendered. If a copayment is required from the patient and you attempt to save and exit the Transaction Entry screen without entering a copayment amount, a reminder notice will appear. This reminder notice gives you the option of returning to the entry screen and entering the copayment amount, or saving without collecting the copayment.

Annual Deductible: This field shows the amount of the annual deductible. This information was entered in the policy information screens in the Patients/Guarantors list.

OA: Other Arrangements. If anything had been entered in the Other Arrangements field of the Patients/Guarantors List, that information would show up here. This is to remind you of any special arrangements which may have been made on this account (i.e., professional courtesy, no charge).

Charges: This field shows the total of all charges entered at this time.

Adjustments: This field shows the total of all adjustments entered at this time.

Subtotal: This field shows a subtotal of the charges and adjustments entered at this time.

Payment: This field shows a total of all payments entered at this time.

Balance: This field shows the result of the subtotal minus the payments.

Account Total: This field shows the result of the balance, plus any remaining balance which was previously shown on this account.

Once you have finished entering transactions you have five options:

1. Update All: will update all transactions entered.

2. Print Receipt: will print the patient a walkout receipt for the charges and payments just entered.

3. Print Claim: will print a CMS-1500 claim form using all entries that have not yet been placed on a claim.

4. Close: will close the transaction window.
5. Save Transactions: will save your input.

Claim Management

The Claim Management screen allows you to select claims that you wish to print or send electronically, reprint, edit, or delete. The first step is to choose the claims which you wish to perform one of the above functions on. Any claims must have previously been entered in the Transaction Entry screen.

Create Claims Screen

Begin by clicking on the **Create Claims** button on the bottom of the claim management screen. This will bring up the Create Claims screen. Here you may choose the transactions you wish to incorporate on a claim by setting the following parameters.

Transaction Dates: Enter the beginning and ending dates of the transactions you wish to work with. You may also click on the calendar to choose a date. This can be helpful if you are unsure of the number of days in a month (i.e., 30 or 31).

Chart Numbers: Enter the beginning and ending chart numbers of the transactions you wish to work with. If you are unsure of the chart numbers, you may click on the magnifying glass to search for a specific number. If you wish to work with only one chart number, enter the same number in both the beginning and ending fields.

Select Transactions That Match: This section allows you to be more specific in your parameters.

Primary Insurance: Enter the Insurance Carrier code. You can enter multiple codes by placing a comma between each code. Leave the space blank to indicate all carriers.

Billing Codes: Enter the billing code. You can enter multiple billing codes by placing a comma between each code. Leave the space blank to indicate all codes.

Case Indicator: Enter the case indicator (i.e., case 1). You can enter multiple case indicators by placing a comma between each one. Leave the space blank to indicate all case indicators.

Location: Enter the location code (place where services were performed). You can enter multiple location codes by placing a comma between each one. Leave the space blank to indicate all location codes.

Provider: Enter the provider code. You can enter multiple provider codes by placing a comma between each one. Leave the space blank to indicate all providers. Indicate whether the provider is Assigned or Attending.

Include transactions if the sum is greater than: This option allows you to create claims for transactions with a specific minimum total dollar amount.

Enter amount: Enter a minimum total amount for a case.

Once you have chosen the parameters, MediSoft will take all transactions which meet these parameters and lump them together on a claim. Therefore, if you have chosen to create a claim for one patient, and that patient has current transactions, but also previous transactions that have not yet been billed, MediSoft will place all open transactions on a single claim and bill them together.

Because of this, it is important that you create claims which match each other. For example, if a patient has two cases, one for a Workers' Compensation injury and one for their regular treatment, you will need to first create a claim for their regular treatment and then create a new claim for their Workers' Compensation treatment, since you cannot bill for both types of services on the same claim.

Once you have created the claim(s), you may choose to perform one of the following functions:

1. Edit the information on the claim by clicking on the **Edit** button.
2. Print a paper claim and/or send an electronic claim.
3. Reprint the claim.
4. Delete the claim.

Edit Claim Icon Option

This option allows you to change data on the claim you have already created. There are five types of changes you can make:

1. Changes to the information for carrier 1.
2. Changes to the information for carrier 2.
3. Changes to the information for carrier 3.
4. Changes to the transaction.
5. Add comments to the claim.

Carrier 1, 2, and 3 Screens

These screens are used for entering information on the insurance carrier

Claim Status: These fields help to track each claim. Once a claim has been completed with all appropriate information, the computer will mark it "Ready to Send." If you wish to change the status of the claim, you may do so here. Your choices are:

Hold the claim to Print/Send at a future date.

Ready to Send.

Sent (once a claim has been sent electronically, the MediSoft program will indicate this). If you are printing claims and sending them in on paper, you will need to manually click on this item when a claim has been sent.

Rejected indicates that the claim was rejected by the insurance carrier or by the clearinghouse.

Challenge indicates that you are or will be appealing the rejection of the claim.

Alert is used to indicate when something is wrong on the claim and further research may need to be done (i.e., no word has been received from the insurance carrier for an extended period of time).

Done indicates that the claim has been paid by the insurance carrier. Some offices will not mark a claim as done until the patient has paid their portion of the claim and the claim has a zero balance.

Pending indicates that the claim is being pended or held until further information is received from the provider or the patient.

Billing Method: This section allows you to choose whether to send a claim on paper or electronically. For example, if you normally send claims electronically, you may want to print out and send manually a claim which needs several pages of documentation.

Batch/Submission Count: The MediSoft program will automatically batch together claims which are sent and will indicate the batch number here, along with the number of claims included in the batch.

Billing Date: This box allows you to indicate the date on which these claims were billed. This can help track how long it has been since a claim was submitted, and whether or not you need to follow-up with the insurance carrier.

Insurance 1: This box will indicate the primary insurance carrier associated with this claim(s).

EDI/EMC Receiver: This box allows you to change the entity (i.e., clearinghouse) which will be receiving this claim.

Transactions Screen

This screen allows you to edit the transactions which appear on this claim.

Comment Screen

This screen allows you to add a comment or additional documentation regarding this claim or the sending of this claim.

Print/Send Claims Icon Option

This option allows you to print paper claims and/or send electronic claims. Upon clicking on the choice, you will be given the option of printing paper claims or sending electronic claims. Only one choice may be done at a time. If you are choosing to send electronic claims, you may choose the receiver to whom you are sending the claims. If you are sending claims to more than one receiver, you will need to complete the sending of claims to one receiver, and then choose to print claims for a second receiver.

Often provider offices will choose to send claims to only one clearinghouse. However, even if a clearinghouse has been chosen, there may be a few insurance carriers who wish to have claims submitted directly to them.

Reprint Claim Icon Option

This screen allows you to reprint a claim which has already been printed. Upon clicking on this choice, you will be asked for the proper format of the claim you wish to reprint, or the carrier you wish to reprint the claim for. This choice is most often used when there are several carriers on a claim and you need to print a separate claim for each carrier, or when a claim has been lost or misplaced and needs to be resubmitted.

Delete Claim Icon Option

This will delete a claim which you have just created. Thus, any transactions which were associated with this claim will be released and you may then choose to create a different claim using these transactions.

Summary

The Activities Menu option includes the Enter Transaction screens and the Claim Management screens. Most activities involving the patient occur in the Transaction Entry screen. This is where all charges, payments, and adjustments are entered into the system. The Claim Management screens allow you to create and print or send claims as well as edit the claims.

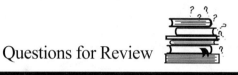

Questions for Review

Directions: Answer the following questions without looking back into the material just covered. Write your answers in the space provided.

1. What items are entered through the Transaction Entry screen? _____

2. List 2 reasons you want to reprint a claim.

    1. _____
    2. _____

3. How do you end an entry in the Charge Entry screen? _____

4. What are the five types of changes you can make to a claim you have created?

    1. _____
    2. _____
    3. _____
    4. _____
    5. _____

5. Once you have finished entering transactions, what are your five options?

    1. _____
    2. _____
    3. _____
    4. _____
    5. _____

If you were unable to answer any of the questions, refer back to that section, and then fill in the answers.

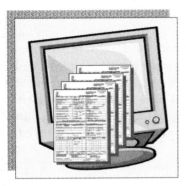

8

Reports Menu Options

After completion of this chapter you will be able to:

- Identify and create various reports.
- Print reports.

The Reports Menu option allows you to print reports to assist in the running of the office and analyzing the practice's accounts. It includes options such as printing patient day sheets; procedure day sheets; payments day sheets; patient ledgers; patient aging; practice analysis; primary, secondary, and tertiary insurance aging; and patient statements. There is also an option for custom reports (i.e., patient lists, address lists, etc.) and for designing your own reports and bills.

Upon choosing many of the options in this list, you will be presented with a window which asks "Print Report Where?" Your three selections are:
1. Preview the report on the screen,
2. Print the report on the printer, and
3. Export the report to a file.

Choose the option you prefer. If desired, you can preview the report on the screen and then print it to the printer.

Once you have chosen one of the above options, click on **Start** to begin the printing process or **Cancel** to take you out of the Reports Menu. If you choose Start you will be taken into a second

screen which allows you to set the parameters for the reports by asking certain questions.

Sort Questions

Since most options present you with the same screen, we will list the questions which may appear on the various screens, then describe each screen and its purpose. These questions help to limit the report to the items you want, rather than including everything. Note that if you do not enter any information in the given field, it indicates there is no limitation for the search and all records will be included.

Some fields will appear on some screens, but not others. Additionally, some of these fields will appear on some versions of MediSoft, but not others. To print reports, simply complete the fields found in your version, and then choose the option to print.

Chart Number Range: Enter the range of the chart numbers you wish to print. Chart numbers are sorted alphabetically. Pressing Enter will include all chart numbers. If you wish to print a ledger for a single person, enter the patient's chart number in both the beginning and ending positions (i.e., ANDAD010-ANDAD010).

Date Created Range: Enter the from and to dates for which the report was created.

Date From Range: Enter the beginning and ending dates which you want included on the report.

Attending Provider Range: Enter the range of provider codes for the providers you would like included in this report. Providers are chosen according to their placement in the Provider List. Pressing Enter will include all providers.

Patient Billing Code Range: If you only wish to include patients within certain billing codes, enter the range of billing codes here. This item corresponds with the Billing Codes which were entered in the Billing Codes List. This allows you to limit patients to those in a certain billing cycle or billed during a certain time of month. To include all patients, press Enter.

Patient Indicator Match: This field refers to the Patient Indicator field which was used in the Patient Information Account screen. Using patient indicators in conjunction with billing codes can create a wide range of printing possibilities. For example, if you wanted to indicate all patients with a certain diagnosis, this diagnosis could be used as an indicator. Thus, you could print all patients with a certain diagnosis who are billed during the first week of the month.

Code 1 Range: Enter the range of the codes from the Procedure/Payment/Adjustments List which you would like included in the report. This option allows you to limit your report to certain types of procedures. For example, entering 99201 to 99215 will limit the report to all office visits.

Patient Reference Balance Range: This field allows you to limit the report to only those patients who have an outstanding balance on their account. Enter the beginning and ending range of the balances you would like to print with no decimal or cents amount. For example, you may want to print only those patients who have a balance of more than $5 but less than $100 (i.e., 5 to 100). To print $5 and above, enter 5 to 999999. If you leave this field blank, the report will show all families, whether they have current transactions and balances or not.

Insurance Carrier 1, 2, or 3 Range: Enter a range of insurance carrier codes. The code refers to the insurance code entered in the Insurance Information screen. The 1, 2 or 3 indicates whether the carriers pay as primary, secondary or tertiary on the claim.

Primary/Secondary Billing Date Range: Enter the beginning and ending dates you want included on the report. Primary refers to the first date for which the claim was billed. Secondary refers to the date this claim was first submitted to the secondary insurance carrier.

Patient Type Range: Enter the types of patients you would like included in the report. These patients can be sorted to include only those covered by Medicare, Medicaid or group insurance.

Preview Screen Icons

Once you preview a report on the screen, a new set of icons will appear across the top of the page. These icons can help you to view the report more easily, and to move quickly among the different pages of a report. The presence of certain icons will depend on which version of MediSoft you are using.

There are three sizes which the report can be shown on the screen. To change the size of the report, click on one of the first three icons at the top left of the page.

The **first icon** will make the report fit within the size of your screen. The **second icon** will enlarge the picture to 100% of what would print. Since most screens are less than 8.5 by 11 inches, this means that a portion of the report will be off the sides and the top or bottom of the screen.

The **third icon** will enlarge the report so that its width is the same width as your screen. This allows you to see more detail, but some items will be scrolled off the top or the bottom of the page.

The ◄ **and** ► **keys** will move you through the various pages of the reports. The first one will return you to the first page in the document. The second will move you back one page. The third one will move you forward one page, and the last one will move you to the last page of the report. Most appointment lists for a single doctor have only one page so these items are not always used with the appointment menu.

The **Printer icon** allows you to print the appointment list from the screen to the printer.

The **Diskette icon** will save the report to a diskette.

The **Folder icon** will load (retrieve) a report which was saved earlier.

The **Close icon** will exit you from the report preview screen.

The **Go To Page box** will allow you to move to a specified page quickly by entering the page number you wish to appear on the screen.

Following are descriptions of each of the different reports and options found under the Reports Menu option.

Day Sheets

A day sheet gives an overview of the provider's day. The **Patient Day Sheet** details the patients seen, showing all transactions and a summary of the day's activities. The **Procedure Day Sheet** details the procedures that were done and shows the patient treated for each procedure. The **Payment Day Sheet** details the money the practice received on that day broken into cash payments, copayments, check payments, and insurance payments; and show the charges to which the payments were applied.

Patient Ledger

A patient ledger records all transactions on a patient's account. It shows the services received, billed amounts, payments, adjustments, and balances. It is useful in noting the activity on each patient's account.

With MediSoft, you can include only those transactions which have not been paid, or all transactions for a given range of dates.

Exercise 8 – 1: Print a patient ledger for Ben Waite. Accept the default setting for all selection questions except Attending Provider Range. Here, you will include only Dr. Phil Goode's patients. Enter the provider code for Dr. Phil Goode in both range areas.

What information is included on the patient ledger?

_____

_____

_____

Patient Aging

A patient aging report allows you to see which patients have outstanding balances and the length of time those balances have been outstanding. This report is most often used when attempting to collect on past due accounts. MediSoft calculates the number of days between the creation of the transaction or claim and the date of the report. The columns break down into 30, 60, 90, and 90+ days old. Since this report is taken from the date the transaction was created (not the date services were rendered) it gives a more accurate picture of how long an account has had an open balance on it. For this reason it is important to enter transactions and create claims as soon after the services were rendered as possible.

Exercise 8 – 2: Print a patient aging report for all patients with balances. Include only Dr. Phil Goode's clients.

List some of the items included on a Patient Aging Report?

_____

_____

_____

_____

_____

Practice Analysis

This report prints the procedures done during a specified period, the amount charged, quantity performed, and the costs and net amount received for each code. It allows the practice to see the types of procedures they are performing and the net receipts from those services. Some practices use this report in creating their monthly financial statements.

Exercise 8 – 3: Print a practice analysis with all procedure codes, dates, and providers.

Ⓠ What information is included on the Practice Analysis Report?

_____

_____

_____

Primary/Secondary/Tertiary Insurance Aging

Insurance Aging Reports allow a practice to see the age of those claims that have been submitted to insurance carriers for payment. Reports are sorted by insurance carrier, thus allowing a biller to see all claims which are owed by a single carrier. Patients who have both primary and secondary insurance will appear on two reports, one for each carrier. As with the Patient Aging Report, Insurance Aging Reports calculate the age of the claim by the number of days between the time the transaction was entered and the date the report was printed. Entries are then separated into 30, 60, 90, 120, and 120+ columns.

Below each patient listed, a tally line appears showing the totals in each aging column both for that patient and for the insurance carrier. The insurance carrier's portion is calculated by multiplying the patient's amount times the percentage of insurance coverage (i.e., 80% in and 80/20 plan).

Exercise 8 – 4: View on the screen an insurance aging report for all primary insurances. Include all dates and all providers.

Ⓠ List some of the items included on an Insurance Aging Report?

_____

_____

_____

_____

Patient Statements

Patient Statements are sent to patients every month to give them a record of their visits and the payments on those visits. They are used by many practices as a monthly bill for patients.

MediSoft allows you several different types of patient statements: a Patient Statement (30, 60, 90), a Patient statement (Color) (one in color), Patient Statement (Color) (30, 60, 90), Patient Statement (with charges only), a Pre-Printed Statement (with the text only, without lines or color so you can print it on a preprinted statement form), a Sample Statement with Image, and a Sample Statement with Logo. You are also given the option of showing file names.

Exercise 8 – 5: Preview patient statements on the screen. Choose the Patient Statement report title (not color or pre-printed). Choose all charts, dates, billing code ranges, indicator ranges, and patient types. It may take a moment to generate this report. After viewing the report, print the statement for Ben Waite by going to the page showing his statement. Click on the printer icon at the top of the screen. Choose the Pages Print Range and enter the page number for Ben Waite's statement (from the upper-right corner of the screen).

Ⓠ List some of the items included on a Patient Statement?

_____

_____

_____

Custom Report List

MediSoft has created a number of custom reports. Most of these include lists of the data entered into the Lists menu option. These lists have been created by MediSoft. To print a list, click on the type of list you would like to print, and then click on **OK**.

Exercise 8 – 6: Print a Patient List for all patients in the practice.

What information is included on a Patient List?

_____

_____

_____

_____

_____

_____

Load Saved Reports: This option allows you to reopen reports that were prepared earlier and were saved.

Design Custom Reports and Bills

With this option, MediSoft allows you to create your own customized reports and bills. Each practice can design a specific report, letter, or document with data imported from the lists, or any specific portion of the list. Since most practices have already created their own reports, and this option takes a tremendous amount of practice and knowledge of report layout and custom designing skills, we will not discuss the creation of new reports in this text. If you wish to create a customized report, consult your MediSoft Patient Accounting User Manual.

Summary

The Reports Menu option allows you to print reports to assist in the running of the office and analyzing the practice's accounts. It includes options such as printing patient day sheets; procedure day sheets; payment day sheets, patient ledgers; patient aging, practice analysis; primary, secondary, and tertiary insurance aging; and patient statements. There is also an option for custom reports (i.e., patient lists, address lists, etc.) and for designing your own reports and bills.

For each report, you have the option of displaying the report on the screen or printing it to paper.

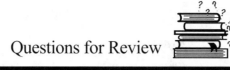

Questions for Review

Directions: Answer the following questions without looking back into the material just covered. Write your answers in the space provided.

1. What information is included on the Patient Ledger? _____

    _____

2. What is the purpose of the Insurance Aging Report? _____

    _____

    _____

3. What information is included on a Patient Day Sheet? _____

    _____

4. What information is included on a Practice Analysis? _____

    _____

    _____

5. How do you preview a report on the screen? _____

    _____

If you were unable to answer any of the questions, refer back to that section, and then fill in the answers.

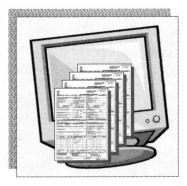

9

Edit, Tools, Window, and Help Menus

After completion of this chapter you will be able to:

- Demonstrate use of the Edit and Tools menu options.
- Access the Help menu to assist in using the MediSoft program.

The items within the Edit, Tools, Window, and Help Menus are not as extensive and thus, we will deal with all of them in this chapter.

Edit Menu Options

The Edit Menu option deals primarily with the handling of text, often in specific windows. By using your mouse to highlight a portion of the text you may choose to perform any of the following options. To highlight a portion of text, use your mouse to position the cursor at the beginning of the text which you wish to cut, copy, or delete. Then, while holding down the left mouse button, move the cursor to the end of the text you wish to modify. Once the text is highlighted, choose one of the following options:

Cut the highlighted portion of the text. This is most often done when you wish to move a portion of the text from one area to another. To move text you would first highlight it, and then click on Cut.

You would then move the cursor to where you wish to insert the text and use the paste option.

Copy the highlighted portion of the text. First highlight the portion of the text you wish to copy. Then click on the Copy option. Then move your cursor to the position where you wish the text to be copied, and click again.

Paste the highlighted portion of the text. This option inserts the portion of text that was last cut into the current position of the cursor.

Delete the highlighted portion of the text. Once a portion of text has been highlighted, by clicking on this option, the highlighted portion of the text will be erased.

Using these options will allow you to modify your text faster than if you were to use the delete keys and/or type in the information again.

Tools Menu Options

The Tools Menu option allows you to look up information regarding your system and its setup, as well as to use an on screen calculator.

The **Calculator** within the MediSoft system works the same as a normal desktop calculator. It can perform addition, subtraction, multiplication, and division functions, as well as calculate percents and square roots. You can use your numeric keypad to enter numbers and operations into the calculator (with the Num Lock on), or you can use your mouse to choose numbers and functions. This tool can be especially useful when performing transaction entries.

The **View File** option allows you to open and view an existing file which has previously been saved.

The **Add/Copy User Reports** option allows you to add or copy reports which you have created.

The **Customize Menu Bar** option allows you to change the icons that appear on your system or the menu bars that appear at the side of your screen.

Choosing the **System Information** option will bring up information regarding your system, including which version of Windows and DOS you are using, how much space you have available in your computer, and the type of printer you are using. This screen is for informational purposes only. Nothing can be edited here.

The **Modem Check** option allows you to test your modem to see if it is working. Since we are not sending items electronically, we will not be using this menu option.

The **User Information** option creates a User Information Report. This report details the name and address of the practice, its phone number, tax ID number, as well as other data.

Exercise 9 – 1: Preview a User Information Report on the screen by clicking on the User Information option, then choosing preview the report on the screen, then click on Start.

List some of the information included in the User Information Report?

_____

_____

_____

_____

_____

The following menu option does not appear in the 2004 MediSoft version but may appear in earlier versions of the software:

The **MediSoft Terminal** menu option can be used to send or receive various reports by connecting to various bulletin boards using a modem. A Bulletin Board System (BBS) is a system which can provide you with information regarding the status of your claims. Since we are not equipped to send claims electronically, we will not be using this option.

Window Menu Options

The Window Menu option allows you to move quickly between the windows you have open. For example, if you open the Patient List, then choose a patient, you have two windows open. You can click back and forth between them by using this option and simply clicking on the window you wish to view. Each time you open a new window, that window will appear superimposed over the existing window. All windows remain open until you click on the icon in the upper-left corner and choose Close to close them, or click on the red X in the upper-right corner.

This menu option also allows you to quickly close all of the windows you have open by clicking on the Close All Windows option.

Help Menu Options

The Help Menu option provides you with information regarding the MediSoft system and how to use it. By clicking on this menu option you can perform the following functions:

Bring up a **Table of Contents** which will tell you about any topic, how to access it, and/or how to perform the function (i.e., how to enter a new patient). The Table of Contents can provide you with an easy reference tool if you forget how to accomplish a task in MediSoft.

The **How to Use Help** option brings up basic instructions on all the options available to you through the Help Menu option. There are numerous topics listed which you can read about by simply clicking on the topic.

It is also possible to print the information which you look up in the Table of Contents and How to Use Help screens by looking up the information on the screen, then clicking on the File menu option in the upper-left corner, and choosing Print Topic.

The **Upgraders from NDCMediSoft for DOS** option provides instructions and tips for those people who have been using a DOS based system and have files entered into the MediSoft for DOS system which they wish to have copied into the MediSoft for Windows system. Converting these files from DOS to Windows can save tremendous amounts of time since each patient and their history (previous transactions) will not have to be re-entered.

The **NDCMediSoft on the Web** option is a link to various internet pages containing pertinent information regarding the MediSoft software.

The **Show Hints** option is an on/off key. If you wish MediSoft to provide you with hints on how to complete many of the fields in the MediSoft screen, click on this option. A check by the option means the hints will be shown. No check means the hints will not be shown.

The **Show Shortcut Keys** tells the MediSoft program whether or not you would like to see the short-cut keys to perform a function (usually Alt combined with a letter). A check by the option means the shortcut keys will be shown. No check means the shortcut keys will not be shown.

Each MediSoft program must be registered within 90 days of activation or the purchaser will be locked out of the program. The **Register Program** option provides you with the registration form which must be completed in order to register your program.

The **About NDCMediSoft** option provides you with the version number of the MediSoft program you are currently working in and whether it is a single-user version or one designed to be networked.

Summary

The Edit Menu option deals primarily with the handling of text, often in specific windows. By using your mouse to highlight a portion of the text you may choose to cut, copy, paste, or delete a portion of text.

The Tools Menu option allows you to look up information regarding your system and its setup, as well as to use an on-screen calculator.

The Windows Menu option allows you to move quickly between the windows you have open. It also allows you to quickly close all of the windows you have open by clicking on the Close All Windows option.

The Help Menu option provides you with information regarding the MediSoft system and how to use it.

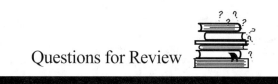

Questions for Review

Directions: Answer the following questions without looking back into the material just covered. Write your answers in the space provided.

1. What four options are available in the Edit Menu?

    1. _____

    2. _____

    3. _____

    4. _____

2. What does the Tools Menu option allow you to do? _____

    _____

    _____

3. What is the purpose of the View File option? _____

    _____

4. How do you access the MediSoft calculator? _____

    _____

5. List the five options available under the Window Menu options.

    1. _____

    2. _____

    3. _____

    4. _____

    5. _____

If you were unable to answer any of the questions, refer back to that section, and then fill in the answers.

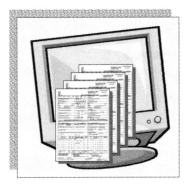

10

Office Hours
Menu Options

After completion of this chapter you will be able to:

- Access the Office Hours Main Menu options.
- Set recurring appointments and breaks.
- Change the program options and create a customized appointment list.

Choosing the Appointment Book option under the Patient Management sidebar opens the Office Hours program. Office Hours is a separate scheduling and time management program. This program makes scheduling appointments simple and easy with just the use of a few key strokes allowing you to enter, change, and delete patient appointments. You may also enter the Office Hours program through the main windows screen by choosing the Office Hours icon rather than the MediSoft program icon.

Menu options for the Office Hours program allows you to perform all necessary functions for setting up and tracking patient appointments.

Office Hours Main Menu Options

As with the MediSoft program, there are several main menu options which occur across the top of the screen. Clicking on a main menu option will bring up a list of submenu options which you may choose from. There are eight main menu options in the Office Hours program:

1. File
2. Edit
3. Search
4. View
5. Lists
6. Reports
7. Tools
8. Help

The **File Menu** option allows you to perform the following functions:

1. Open Practice
2. New Practice
3. Program Options
4. File Maintenance
5. Backup Data
6. Restore Data
7. Exit

The **Edit Menu** option allows you to perform what functions?

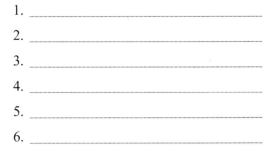

1. _____
2. _____
3. _____
4. _____
5. _____
6. _____

7. _____

8. _____

The **View Menu** option allows you to perform what functions?

1. _____

2. _____

3. _____

4. _____

5. _____

6. _____

7. _____

8. _____

The **Lists Menu** option allows you to perform what functions?

1. _____

2. _____

3. _____

4. _____

5. _____

6. _____

The **Reports Menu** option allows you to perform what functions?

1. _____

2. _____

a. _____

3. _____

4. _____

5. _____

6. _____

7. _____

The **Tools Menu** option allows you to perform what function?

1. _____

The **Help Menu** option allows you to perform what functions?

1. _____

2. _____

3. _____

4. _____

a. _____

b. _____

c. _____

d. _____

e. _____

5. _____

6. _____

File Menu Options

The File Menu option is the first main menu option, and it allows you to perform the following functions:

1. Open Practice
2. New Practice
3. Program Options
4. File Maintenance
5. Backup Data
6. Restore Data
7. Exit

Open Practice

This option allows you to open (retrieve) the data that has been stored regarding this practice. This includes data both about the practice and about the individual appointments which have been set up for that practice.

New Practice

This option allows you to create a new set of data for setting up appointments. If you have set up your practice using the MediSoft program File Menu, that data will already have been created and you will not need to create a new set of data.

If you have not previously set up data, enter the name of the doctor or practice, and then enter the data path where you would like this information to be stored.

Program Options

The program options file menu allows you to customize the appointment lists and reports in these ways:

1. The starting and ending time for the practice.
2. The number of minutes between each listed time (i.e., every half hour instead of every 15 minutes).
3. The number of booking columns (if your office has several treatment rooms).
4. Default Colors for Appointments, Scheduling Conflicts, and Breaks.

You can also specify whether you want the following options enabled or disabled:

1. Use Enter to move between fields.
2. Use automatic word capitalization.
3. Automatic Refresh.
4. Show notes on new appointment.

File Maintenance

Here you have the same File Maintenance options which appear in the MediSoft File Maintenance menu. However, these apply only to the data which has been entered into the Office Hours program (i.e., Appointment Lists, Patient Lists, and Provider Lists.) You may choose to rebuild these lists, pack them, backup data, purge data, or restore data. For additional information, see the File Maintenance options in Chapter 4.

Exit

This option allows you to exit the Office Hours program. If you entered the Office Hours program through the MediSoft Activities menu option, you will be returned to the MediSoft program.

Edit Menu Options

The Edit Menu option allows you to perform the following functions:

1. Cut
2. Paste
3. Copy
4. Delete
5. Go to Today
6. Go to Date
7. Find Open Time
8. Find Next Open Time

This allows you to cut, copy, paste, delete, and find appointments.

Cut allows you to cut an appointment. This is most often done when you wish to move an appointment from one time to another or from one date to another. To move an appointment, you would first highlight it, and then click on **Cut**. You would then use the mouse to move the cursor to where you wish to insert the appointment by changing the date (if necessary), then use the Paste option to insert the information.

Copy allows you to copy an appointment. First highlight the appointment you wish to copy. Then click on the **Copy** option. Then move your cursor to the position where you wish the appointment to be copied, and click again. This option is most often used when a patient is setting up two or more appointments. Using this option prevents you from having to re-enter the patient information each time.

Paste allows you to insert the appointment that was last cut into the current position of the cursor. It is used with Cut to move an appointment from one place to another.

Delete allows you to quickly delete an appointment. By clicking on this option, the highlighted appointment will be erased.

Using these options allows you to modify your appointment schedules faster than if you were to use the delete keys and/or type in the information again.

Go To Today allows you to quickly see appointments entered for today.

The **Go To Date** menu option allows you to quickly move from one date to another. After clicking on this option, you may choose to go to a specific date if it is known. There are also options for going to a date that is a specified number of days, weeks, months, or years from the current year. This is used when the provider requests that the patient return in a specified period of time (i.e., two weeks) for a follow-up appointment. The years option is seldom used, however, providers who treat cancer patients may mark a date five years from the date the cancer is in remission (a patient may be considered cured if he is cancer free for five years) or patients can easily be scheduled for a yearly check-up using this option.

The **Find Open Time** option searches for available time slots in a provider's schedule. Fill in the length of the appointment and its start and end time and click on the day of the week you wish to schedule an appointment for and click **Search**. The program will display the time slot and show you if anything has been scheduled for that time and day.

The **Find Next Open Time** option allows you to search again if the first date was unacceptable for any reason.

View Menu Options

The view menu option allows you to indicate whether or not you would like the **calendar**, **status bar** and/or **tool bar** to appear on the screen. A check mark beside each option indicates it is viewable on the screen. No check mark indicates it is not.

You can also **Zoom in** or **Zoom out** on the screen.

The **Refresh** option redraws the information on your screen so it appears properly. Otherwise data on the screen may seem to overlap.

Lists Menu Options

The Lists Menu option has six submenu options:
1. Appointment List
2. Break List
3. Patient List
4. Provider List
5. Resource List
6. Reason List

The Office Hours program automatically pulls the information in these lists from the Patients/Guarantors List and Providers List in the MediSoft program. These options allow you to edit or add patients, guarantors, providers, and staff members to the existing lists. The information which is added or changed here will also appear in the corresponding MediSoft list. The data which is entered here is the same as was entered in the MediSoft program. If you need further information on completing these fields, see Chapters 5 and 6.

Here you also have the opportunity to create lists of breaks, resources, and reasons. Breaks are items such as lunch or coffee breaks which may need to be scheduled into a provider's day. Resources are the rooms available for use (i.e., two exam rooms, a conference room, lunch room, etc.). Reasons are the reason a patient may be requesting

an appointment or the type of patient they are (i.e., Medicare patient).

Reports Menu Options

The reports menu options allow you to print reports. The choices in this menu option include printing:

Appointment List: This option prints a list of appointments that have been scheduled.

Print Appointment Grid: This prints a list of appointments in grid format.

Print Superbills: This feature allows you to print superbills for patients. Superbills allow providers to quickly report the services performed and their diagnoses.

Reasons: Is a list of the reasons which have been entered into the computer.

Custom Report List: Is a list of all the custom reports that have been created by the practice.

Load Saved Reports: Allows you to load reports you may have previously saved.

Design Custom Reports and Bills: Allows you to create a report that has just what you want in it.

Once you have chosen any of these reports, you will be asked whether you want the report printed to the screen, to a file, or to the printer. If you choose to send the report to the screen you will still have the option of printing it after you view it.

Once you have chosen where the report will be sent, a new screen will allow you to choose the parameters. This is most often the date, provider, or chart (patient).

Tools Menu Options

The Tools Menu option contains the **System Information**. This option will bring up information about your system, including which version of Windows and DOS you are using, how much space you have available in your computer, and the type of printer you are using. This screen is for informational purposes only.

Help Menu Options

The Help Menu option provides you with information about the MediSoft system and how to use it. By clicking on this menu option you can perform the following functions:

Bring up a **Table of Contents** that will tell you about any topic, how to access it, and/or how to perform the function (i.e., how to enter a new patient). The Table of Contents can provide you with an easy reference tool if you forget how to accomplish a task in MediSoft.

It is also possible to print the information which you look up in the Table of Contents and How to Use Help screens by looking up the information on the screen, then clicking on the File Menu option in the upper-left hand corner, and choosing Print Topic.

The **Show Balloon Hints** option allows you to turn on and off the balloon hints which appear next to a field in which the cursor is placed. A check mark beside this option indicates that the balloon hints will show. Clicking on this option will remove the check mark and the balloon hints will not show. The hints will still appear at the bottom of the page, regardless of whether this option is turned on or off.

Clear Window Positions allows you to take off the window options quickly.

The **NDCMediSoft on the Web** option allows you to immediately connect to the NDCMediSoft website. This item is simply an internet link to their site.

The **Online Updates** option allows you to quickly receive online updates to the software. This is also a link to their website. It should be noted that in order for these options to work, your computer must have Internet access.

Finally, the **About Office Hours** option allows you to view which version of MediSoft you are using.

Search Options

This option is not found in all versions of MediSoft. However, this option allows you to search for information using many variables.

Quick Select Icons

Across the top of the screen are 14 quick select icons. These icons allow you to choose a function to perform without going through the process of selecting a menu option, then selecting a suboption. The quick select icons include:

1. Appointment Entry
2. Break Entry
3. Appointment List
4. Break List
5. Patient List
6. Provider List
7. Resource List
8. Go To Date
9. Search For Open Time Slot
10. Search Again
11. Go To Today
12. Print Report
13. Help
14. Exit

Let's look at each of these in a bit more depth.

Appointment Entry

This option opens a screen for entering information for a new appointment. This will be discussed in more depth in the next chapter.

Break Entry

This option allows you to create breaks in a provider's schedule. These can be either a single break or a recurring daily break in a provider's schedule (i.e., lunch from 12 p.m. to 1 p.m.). On some versions of MediSoft this function was performed by two buttons, a Break Entry and a Recurring Break Entry option.

Appointment List

This option allows you to find an appointment quickly and easily when you do not have all the information on the appointment (i.e., date and time). For example, you can locate a patient's appointment by typing their name into the search field.

To find an appointment, click on this option. When the search window pops up, first choose the data you wish to sort by. Click on the **Search by** field and choose whether you wish to search for an appointment by the chart number, the date of the appointment, the name of the patient, or the provider. Most often it will be easiest to search by the name of the patient. Once you have completed this field, click on the **Search for** field and begin entering the chart number, date of appointment, name of the patient, or the provider. You may enter all or part of the data. When you have entered data into this field, press enter. Any items which match the chart number, date, name or provider will appear in the search window. The date and time of the appointment will also appear to assist you in choosing the one you wish to see. Click on the item you wish to see and the information will appear on the screen. If there is only one appointment which matches the information you have entered in the Search for field, that information will appear on the screen without the use of the search window.

Break List

This option displays a list of all scheduled breaks so you can see when a provider is out of the office.

Patient List

This option shows you a list of the patients currently entered into the system and allows you to edit them. You may also add a new patient using this option. For more information, see the List menu option: Patients/ Guarantors.

Provider List

This option shows you a list of the providers currently entered into the system and allows you to edit current providers or add new ones.

Resource List

This is a list of the rooms that are available. If a provider has more than one exam room, an overlapping appointment can be scheduled in the each of the rooms.

Go To Date

This option allows you to quickly go to a specific date. For more information, see the Edit menu option Go To Date.

Search For Open Time Slot

This allows you to search for time slots that may be open on a specific date or at a specific time.

This can be especially helpful when you are setting up an appointment and the patient is looking for the earliest time the provider can see him or her.

To find available appointment times, click on the **Find** menu option. Enter the length of the appointment which the patient desires or will need. If you are unsure of the amount of time a certain procedure will take, look up the procedure using the appointment scheduling screen in the main menu. Entering a procedure number will allow the length of the appointment to show in the length field directly below the procedure.

Enter the beginning hour and minutes which the patient would consider coming in, then click on a.m. or p.m. to indicate morning or afternoon.

Enter the ending hour and minutes after which the patient is unable to come in, then click on a.m. or p.m. to indicate morning or afternoon. Be sure there is an X next to any days which the patient would consider coming in for the appointment. The Office Hours program automatically enters an X on every day. Therefore, if the patient or the provider would rather not show up on any given days, click on that day and the X will disappear. This is an on/off button, so clicking again will make the X reappear.

Once you have entered the data, click on the word **Search**. The program will automatically find the first available appointment date which meets the criteria which you have entered. If this date is unacceptable for any reason, choose the Search Menu option, and then click on **Search Again**. The program will then go to the next available appointment which meets your criteria.

Search Again

This option allows you to change the parameters and search a second or subsequent time.

Go To Today

Clicking on this icon returns the calendar to the current date.

Print Report

This option prints a copy of the current appointment schedule which is shown on the screen.

Help

This option will allow you to access the help screen.

Exit

This option allows you to exit the Office Hours program. If you entered the Office Hours program through the MediSoft Activities menu option, you will be returned to the MediSoft program.

The following icons may occur in earlier versions of the MediSoft program:

Show/Hide Hints

This is an on/off function key which commands the program to either show or hide the hints which appear in a balloon near the icon or field which the cursor is in.

Summary

The Appointment Book option opens the Office Hours program. This separate MediSoft program which allows you to enter, change, and delete patient appointments. Office Hours program can also be accessed through the main windows screen by choosing the Office Hours icon.

The File Menu option allows you to open a practice, create a practice, backup and restore data, change program options, perform file maintenance, and exit the program.

The Edit Menu options allow you to cut, copy, paste or delete an appointment. The Find Open Time option allows you to quickly find an appointment that was entered. The Go To Date menu option allows you to quickly move from one date to another.

The View, Lists, Reports, Tools, and Help Menu options allow you to select screen display options, retrieve patient and provider information which has been stored, look at the system information for the program you are using, print reports, and ask for help in completing a field or using an option.

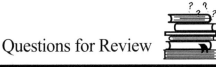

Questions for Review

Directions: Answer the following questions without looking back into the material just covered. Write your answers in the space provided.

1. What menu option allows you to cut and paste data? _____

    _____

2. What menu option allows you to zoom in and out on the screen? _____

    _____

3. What menu option allows you to print out an appointment list? _____

    _____

4. What menu option do you use to find an open time slot? _____

5. What is the purpose of the Break Entry icon? _____

    _____

If you were unable to answer any of the questions, refer back to that section, and then fill in the answers.

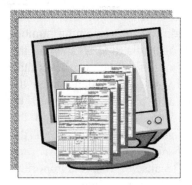

11

Appointment Book

After completion of this chapter you will be able to:

- Set an appointment for a patient.
- Identify and use the quick select icons.

In the chapter we will discuss the Office Hours main screen, the changing of dates and providers, and the entering of appointments.

The Main Screen

The main screen is used for entering appointments on a provider's schedule. Before setting up an appointment, it is important to ensure that you are working on the appointment calendar for the correct provider and are also working on the correct date.

Choosing a Provider
The first step in setting up an appointment is to choose the correct provider. Each provider has their own appointment calendar. You choose the provider you wish to work on by clicking on the Provider Field in the upper -right corner of the screen. This will bring up a list of all the providers who are currently entered into the system. In order for a provider to have an appointment calendar set up, they must have previously been entered into the Provider List screen in either the MediSoft program, or in the Office Hours program (see Provider List for further information).

Choosing a Date
The Office Hours program shows only one date at a time on the screen. In order to properly set appointments, breaks, meetings, or any other items into a provider's schedule, you must be sure that the correct date is showing on the screen.

The Office Hours program will automatically bring up the current date on the screen. To change the date, use the arrows below the calendar on the left of the screen to select the correct date. This will bring up a calendar of the month and year you have chosen. The calendar will show each date on the appropriate day of the month for that month and year. To choose a date, simply click on the date.

Once you have completed these steps, the appointment calendar for the chosen provider on the chosen date will appear on the right half of the screen.

Setting up an Appointment
Setting up an appointment is the most commonly performed function in the Office Hours program.

To set up an appointment for a patient, first be sure you have chosen the correct date and the correct provider. Then double-click on the time you wish to set up an appointment. The Appointment Entry screen will appear. Enter the following information in each of the appointment screen fields:

Exercise 11 – 1: Enter an appointment for Candy Dunnitt on 1/19/XX at 1:30 p.m. with Dr. Phil Goode. She will be having a straightforward office visit and glucose check to monitor her diabetes. Add the message that the patient's weight should be checked during the visit.

Chart/Name: Enter the chart number of the patient. As soon as you begin typing a chart number or name, the automatic search feature will bring up a list of all patients whose chart number matches the letters you have typed. At this point you may click on one of these numbers or names, or continue typing in the complete chart number. You may also use the arrow down to bring up a list of all patients, or the magnifying glass to perform a search for a patient.

Phone: If the patient's phone number was previously entered into the Patient List, it will automatically appear here. If the number is not correct or if the patient can be more easily reached at a different number, enter that number here.

Resource: Enter the location where the appointment will take place. This field has a search option.

Note: Enter any message you wish printed on the appointment list in the space next to the patient's appointment. This can be a reminder for the provider to check the patient's weight or blood pressure, or something more personal such as asking about a family member (i.e., son Bob has cancer). As you type, some characters will scroll off the left side of the field, but they will still print on the appointment list.

Case: If there is more than one case associated with this patient; choose the appropriate case for this visit.

Reason: Enter the reason the patient is requesting the appointment.

Length: Enter the number of minutes the procedure is expected to take. If the procedure takes longer than a single space (usually 15 minutes in length),

then the Office Hours program will place the patient's name in the time slot for the first 15 minutes, and will shade out the remaining number of minutes to indicate that this time is taken by the above patient. Shading is done in 15-minute intervals. Therefore, if you have a patient with a 40-minute appointment, the patient's name will be shown in the first 15-minute time slot, and the following time slot only will be shaded. If the appointment is for 45 minutes, two additional time slots will be shaded. Because of this, it is important to schedule patients in 15-minute intervals. If you wish to change the amount of time in each appointment interval, use the File menu option, click on Program Options and alter the interval (see File Menu options for additional information).

Date: Enter the desired date of the appointment.

Time: Enter the time of the appointment.

Provider: Enter the name of the provider who will be seeing the patient for this appointment.

Repeat: This option allows you to set up multiple appointments at a single time. For example, if a woman is pregnant, she may need to see the doctor every month. If she would like an appointment on the 5th day of every month at the same time, the repeat option can be used to choose a monthly appointment time. Repeat options include daily, weekly, monthly and yearly options. Repeat appointments may also be used to block out a provider's schedule. For example, if the provider has a meeting at the same time every week, this function can block out that time every week.

Change: Clicking this button allows you to set up and/or change the frequency of the repeat appointments.

Procedure Code: This field is not present in the 2004 version of MediSoft, but it may be present in earlier versions. Enter the procedure code for the service which the provider will be performing. This code should previously have been entered in the Procedure Code List in MediSoft. If not, you will need to add it there before entering it here. You may also use the arrow down to bring up a list of all procedure codes, or the magnifying glass to perform a search for a procedure code. If a time was included when the procedure code was entered, the appropriate amount of time would be scheduled for the visit.

After you have completed the above fields, clicking **Save** will place the appointment into the appointment calendar and save the information.

Summary

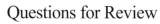

You have now completed the tutorial part of the MediSoft Training Program. You should now have a good working knowledge of the MediSoft Patient Billing software program. However, many things take practice to learn. The following Simulated Work portion of the training program will give you practice entering information in the previously mentioned screens, running reports, and performing all the necessary tasks of a medical biller.

You will have the opportunity to enter numerous patients, as well as claims, payments, appointments, and other activities. By the end of the Simulated Work Program you should be proficient not only in the use of the MediSoft Patient Accounting Program, but in many of the daily tasks of medical billing.

Questions for Review

Directions: Answer the following questions without looking back into the material just covered. Write your answers in the space provided.

1. Before you enter an appointment, be sure you have chosen the correct _____ and

    _____.

2. How do you choose the time you wish to set up an appointment? _____

    _____

3. What is the purpose of the Resource field? _____

    _____

4. What information is entered in the Reason field? _____

    _____

5. What is the purpose of the Repeat field? _____

    _____

If you were unable to answer any of the questions, refer back to that section, and then fill in the answers.

Simulated Work
Program

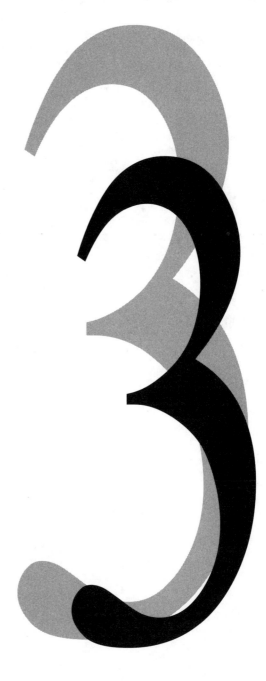

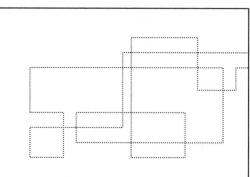

SIMULATED WORK PROGRAM

Congratulations on making it through the tutorial portion. Now you are ready to step into the shoes of a real medical biller and enter a simulated work program.

As a medical biller, it is your job to enter new patients into the system (computerized or manual), bill for services rendered, and keep an accurate log of the provider's accounts. Often you will be required to enter a new doctor or patient into the system. Other times the doctor or patient will already be in the system, and you must locate his or her existing records.

In an actual office setting, doctors will submit numerous patient charge slips, usually one for each patient seen. A doctor can see 20 to 30 patients in an average day, which means creating 20 to 30 patient billings and updating their charts every day. Add in phone calls, dealing with patients, handling mail, receiving payments, and rebilling secondary insurance or patients for any balances left, and you can see how busy the job can become.

This simulated work program is set up to give you practical knowledge in the day-to-day activities of the medical biller. It simulates many of the duties you will be asked to perform in an office setting. Additionally, you will have the opportunity to code and bill numerous types of claims, including physician's services, lab, surgery, assistant surgery, anesthesia, durable medical equipment, and ambulance claims. During this simulated work program be sure to use the dates indicated in the text. **In each case the year 20XX or XX should be replaced with the current year. The year PY should be replaced with the prior year (i.e., if you are completing this in 2004, XX = 2004 and PY = 2003).**

Feel free to use other available resources to complete the assignments. On the job you will often have many of these resources available to you. These can include CPTs®, ICD-9s, medical dictionaries, medical terminology books, medical billing instruction books, reference books on completing forms, etc. If you have difficulty remembering how to complete a screen, do not hesitate to consult the manual that describes the data entry.

In a normal office, only one or perhaps two people in a family will seek treatment. Then an extended period of time elapses before treatment is again sought (unless a chronic condition exists). We have compressed several visits into a three-month period to allow you to gain experience compiling charts, figuring deductibles paid, and seeing how one claim may impact others in a family group. As such, the simulated work program covers five days which are spread throughout this three-month period. When beginning a new day's work, be sure to change the computer to the correct date. Otherwise, data may be posted incorrectly or appear incorrectly on day sheets and other reports.

Additionally, we have limited the scenarios to 14 families so you do not have to enter an excessive number of providers or unrelated patients.

In order to save paper and printing costs, we have summarized the information contained on charge slips rather than presenting the entire charge slip. Likewise, we have included information on dependents on the same form as the insured. This prevents duplication of items such as address, phone number, insurance plan information, etc.

Go through the exercises step by step. Do not skip any or move on until you have fully completed a step. Otherwise your totals on subsequent exercises may be incorrect. The exception to this is for those who have completed the tutorial portion in section 2 of this text. You may skip items 3 – 7 since they were done at that time.

If you are unsure how to complete a step, refer back to the information contained in the tutorial portion. Some steps will ask you to enter data, create reports, or deal with individuals on the telephone. Most steps will deal directly with data contained in this text, however, it is assumed that you will have previously received training on the basic functions of medical billing (i.e., dealing with patients, record keeping, CPT® and ICD-9 coding, completing claim forms, privacy issues, and medical charting). You will need to rely on this knowledge to complete some exercises.

At the end of each day's steps is a section for recording additional information or other data or confirmation which may be needed. If additional information is needed from a patient or other party, list it here then complete a "Request for Additional Information" form which can be found in the back of the book. The outside margins in this section are wider to allow for note taking, and the exercises are marked with an Item check-off box to help keep track of where you stopped working.

You will also encounter a number of critical thinking exercises. These exercises present you with a situation and ask what you would do. They are intended to help you make the transition from trainee to medical biller. Each situation involves a scenario which you may or may not have had training in or experienced before. Be sure to take time to think about your answer. Often there are pitfalls in a situation which may not be obvious. You should call upon the previous learning you have had in this field and remember all rules and regulations regarding privacy issues, collections, and all other aspects of the job.

Here you will have the time to think through an answer, whereas on the job you may not. Try to place yourself in the situation and respond appropriately. Read through the scenario and then write your response in the space provided.

Critical thinking exercises generally do not impact the data entry for the other assignments. If you are unable to come up with the correct answer, do not worry about it. It will not critically impact subsequent entries. Just make your best guess. At the end of the simulated work program, ask the instructor for the answer to those items which you had difficulty with.

If it is easy for you to respond with the correct answer, GREAT! You have learned how to deal with that situation. If you find that your response has faults, do not worry. These situations will probably be the ones that you remember the most. If so, you will have achieved the purpose of this book and learned from the experience of being a medical biller. Hopefully, this book will give you the practical experience both to apply the training you have had and to think on your feet when presented with a new and unusual situation.

If you are completely stumped, there are clues listed for many of the critical thinking exercises at the back of this section. You should attempt to answer the question on your own, then look up the clue. It may provide you with confirmation of your answer or provide you with additional information for handling the situation.

MANUAL AND COMPUTERIZED ENTRY INSTRUCTIONS

This simulated work program may be used by students who are using a manual or pegboard system, as well as those using any computerized medical billing program.

Specific instructions for completing data manually are indicated with the ☞ symbol. Specific instructions for completing data on a computerized system are indicated by the 🖥 symbol. Use only those instructions that are appropriate for your system. Instructions which are appropriate for all users are not indented behind a symbol.

For example:

1. All students or trainees using the simulated work program should read and utilize data which appears in this format.

    ☞ Only those students or trainees using a manual or pegboard system should use these specific instructions.

    🖥 Only those students or trainees using a computerized medical billing system should use these specific instructions.

ENTERING A CLAIM "INTO THE SYSTEM"

At various times patients will need to be billed for services rendered. On the job the provider will complete a superbill or charge slip for the patient which shows the services performed and the related diagnoses. In order to save paper, the simulated work program will list all of the pertinent information regarding services performed in a brief scenario paragraph. This paragraph will be headed with a **CLAIM NUMBER**. To help keep track of papers for this course, place the appropriate claim number in the upper-right-hand corner of each CMS-1500 created.

To give you practice in coding procedures and diagnoses, the appropriate CPT® and ICD-9 codes have not been listed. To complete the billing on a claim, use the CPT® and ICD-9 books to code the procedure and diagnoses. Unless otherwise indicated, all office visits should be considered established patients. To "enter a claim into the system" means to complete each of the following steps.

☞   a.   Complete a CMS-1500 form for the patient visit. If you are not using two-part CMS forms, write up two forms or make a copy of the CMS-1500 when it is completed. One copy will go in the patient chart, the other will be mailed to the insurance carrier.

b.   Update the patient's chart, including patient ledger cards and patient statements.

c.   If the patient made a payment, create a receipt.

a.   If you have not previously done so, enter the patient and any other family members into the Patient Information database.

b.   Enter the CPT® codes into the Procedure Information screens. Some procedures may have been previously entered using Document 4. If so, these procedures do not need to be reentered. If a procedure has already been entered, the data will appear on the screen when you enter the code into the Procedure Code field.

c.   Enter the ICD-9 codes into the Diagnosis Code Information screen. Some diagnoses may have been previously entered using Document 5. If so, these diagnoses do not need to be reentered. If a diagnosis has already been entered, the data will appear on the screen when you enter the code into the Diagnosis Code field.

d.   Enter the charges as shown on the claim scenarios. If a payment was made, enter the payment and print a walkout receipt before saving the data.

Many computer systems allow you to print out all patient claims which were entered in a single day. For this reason there will be a notation at the end of each day for computerized billing users to print out the CMS-1500s which they have entered for that day. Using two-part CMS-1500 forms is suggested. If you are using one-part forms, print out two copies or make a photocopy of the form after it is completed. One copy of the form will go in the patient file, the second copy will be mailed to the insurance carrier for payment.

GETTING STARTED

You are now ready to start the simulated work program. If you are using computerized billing software, you should first become familiar with it. You need not become proficient as you will get plenty of practice using the program during this portion of the text. However, you should be familiar with how the program operates and the correct screen for entering various pieces of data.

When entering transactions (charges or payments), be sure to tie the payment(s) to the proper charge(s). Doing this allows you to keep track of the amount which has been paid on each visit.

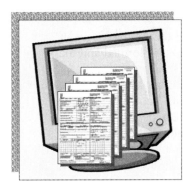

January 14, 20XX

Item 1. ☐ **T**oday's date is January 14, 20XX.

 Change the date to: January 14, 20XX.

Item 2. ☐ **C**ount petty cash. How much is in the cash envelope? _____

Item 3. ☐ **A**t the beginning of each year, your office sends out a patient information sheet to each patient and asks them to complete and return it. This allows the office to keep their information current and ensures that any changes are updated at least yearly. Two patient information sheets arrived in the mail last week (Documents 1 – 2). Review the patient information sheets and create charts for each family and patient. (If you are unsure how to create charts or enter data, refer to the previous chapters.)

> Enter the information from the patient information sheets into the computer. If you previously completed this during section 2 you do not need to re-enter the data.

Item 4. ☐ **Y**ou receive a paper showing the doctors in the CHS family (Document 3).

> ☞ Place Document 3 in an accessible location. This is the list of providers for whom you will be billing and their pertinent information.

> Add the doctors to the Provider Information database. If you previously completed this during section 2 you do not need to re-enter the data.

Item 5. ☐ **A** paper is placed on your desk containing procedure information (Document 4). Look over the information in this document. Note the amount of time each procedure takes. This information may be important when scheduling appointments. Code the procedures.

> ☞ Place Document 4 in an accessible location. This is the list of office visit procedures, with their corresponding allotment and charge information.

Add the procedure information into your system if your system is not using a pre-purchased CPT® code listing. Otherwise, edit the appropriate CPT® code to include the time and standard billing amount. If you previously completed this during section 2 you do not need to re-enter the data.

Item 6. ☐ **A** paper is placed on your desk containing diagnosis information (Document 5). Look over the information in this document and code the diagnoses.

☞ Place Documents in an accessible location.

Add the diagnosis information into your system if your system is not using a pre-purchased ICD-9 code listing. If you previously completed this during section 2 you do not need to re-enter the data.

Item 7. ☐ **T**wo more patient information sheets arrive over the fax machine (Documents 6 – 7). Review the patient information sheets and create charts for each family and patient.

Enter the data from the patient information sheets into the computer.

Item 8. ☐ **Y**ou receive another sheet showing additional doctors in the CHS family (Document 8).

☞ Attach Document 8 to Document 3 and keep both documents in an accessible place.

Add the new doctors to the Provider Information database.

Item 9. ☐ **P**at N. O'Gen saunters up to the billing office window after her son's visit with Dr. Sickman. Enter these charges into the system.

CLAIM 1
Ox O'Gen received a problem focused, straightforward visit performed in the office ($55) today (date of first visit 12/29/PY). Diagnosis: Scarlet Fever, URI.

Item 10. ☐ **S**herry Attricks scuttles up to the window and begins tapping her fingers impatiently on the counter. Behind her, her grandson plops himself into a chair while holding his stomach. Mrs. Attricks hands you a patient information sheet (Document 9) and two charge slips. "I hope this won't take long," she exclaims. "I wasn't planning on scheduling *two* appointments today!" Create a patient and family chart then enter these charges into the system.

CLAIM 2
Petey Attricks received a comprehensive, high complexity exam ($190) in Dr. Phil Goode's office on 1/14/XX. A blood sample was taken ($15). Diagnosis: Abdominal Pain, Gastroenteritis. Petey received an immediate referral to Dr. Ben Dover, Gastroenterologist.

CLAIM 3
Petey Attricks received a new patient comprehensive confirmatory consultation, of moderate complexity performed in the office ($275) by Dr. Ben Dover on 1/14/XX. Patient was referred by Dr. Phil Goode. Diagnosis: Gallstones.

Item
11. ☐ **D**r. Dover prefers to collect the estimated patient portion of the charges at the time of the visit. You call the insurance carrier and find out that Petey has a $125 deductible and none of it has been paid. Insurance pays 80%. Estimate the patient's portion of the charges.

What are the total charges? _____

What is the estimated insurance payment? _____

What is the estimated patient portion? _____

Sherry makes a payment for the above amount with check #1932 (in the Window Payments section behind the documents). Fill in the correct amount on the check. Enter it into the system. Be sure to cut out the check and put it in your petty cash envelope.

Item
12. ☐ **S**herry Attricks also asks for an appointment for herself with Dr. Sickman. Set up an appointment on 1/22/XX at 3:30 p.m. The appointment will take approximately 30 minutes. Use Dr. Sickman's appointment calendar (Document 10).

 Enter the appointment into the computer.

Item
13. ☐ **S**uddenly you look up and there is someone at the window. Codie Pendent smiles at the recognition and hands you the following charge slip information. "My daughter was hurrying to answer the door this morning and tripped and fell," she explains. Enter the charges.

CLAIM 4

Dee Pendent received a minimal service exam in Dr. Goode's office ($35) today. Diagnosis: Multiple Contusions and Abrasions.

Item
14. ☐ **"I**'m feeling a bit overwhelmed with everything lately," Ms. Pendent continues. "I think it might be best to have a visit with the psychiatrist. Do I need authorization for that?" What do you say and do?

_____

_____

_____

_____

Item
15. ☐ **D**r. Phil Goode rushes through the office, late as usual. He drops a bunch of papers on your desk. "I saw these patients at CHS Community Hospital the first half of the month," he explains. "Could you get them into the system as quick as possible? Thanks, bye." He rushes out without waiting for a response.

You leaf through the papers to find three charge slips and some patient information sheets (Documents 11 – 12). Create patient and family charts if needed. Enter these charges into the system.

CLAIM 5

D. Jobb Dunnitt called 911 on 1/9/XX gasping and complaining of chest pain and shortness of breath. Dr. Goode was covering the emergency room at CHS Community Hospital at the time and directed the paramedics in the care of Mr. Dunnitt ($65). When Mr. Dunnitt arrived at the hospital, Dr. Goode performed a comprehensive, high complexity exam ($240). A complete EKG with 12 leads ($140) was given, which determined that there was no heart trouble. An injection of Cleocin was given ($30). Diagnosis: Acute Bronchitis, Chest Pain, Asbestosis.

What additional information is needed from Mr. Dunnitt? _____

_____

CLAIM 6

Mort Allity received a detailed admission performed at CHS Community Hospital ($110) on 1/4/XX. Expanded exams on 1/5, 1/6, and 1/7/XX ($95 each). Patient discharged ($115) on 1/8/XX. Diagnosis: Tonsillopharyngitis.

CLAIM 7

Carla Poole (called "Car" by her friends), an active child involved in soccer, tennis, and skating, was brought to the ER by her mother who stated that she fell while skating at home on 1/8/XX, scraping her knee and cutting her finger. An expanded exam, low complexity was performed at CHS Community Hospital ($55) on 1/8/XX. Car was told to follow-up with her doctor if necessary.

Item
16. ☐ **M**s. Minnie Mumwage, a patient, calls on the phone. "Dr. Goode suggests that I get this complicated course of treatment for my condition, but I can't afford it. There's no way I can pay for this! What do you think I should do?" What do you say?

_____

_____

_____

_____

_____

Item
17. ☐ **S**tu Pididiot comes into the office for his appointment. He thinks he saw a doctor here several years ago but he is not sure which doctor it was.

How would you determine if he is still listed as a patient? _____

_____

Item
18. ☐ **I**ma Knose arrives at the window after her visit with Dr. Goode. She hands you a patient information sheet (Document 13) and charge slips containing the following information. Create a patient and family chart. Enter these charges into the system.

CLAIM 8

Ima Knose received a minimal office visit ($40), an injection of 1/4 cc of Gomenol ($30), and .10cc of Calcium Glucose ($30) given at the office on 1/14/XX. Supplies and materials: $12. Diagnosis: Hypoestrogenism, Hyperlipidemia. A cash payment of $25 was made for this visit (see Window Payments section). Patient requests a receipt.

Item 19. ☐ **D**uring the same visit Ron E. Knose also received treatment. Enter these charges.

CLAIM 9

Ron E. Knose received an expanded exam with history performed by Dr. Phil Goode in the office ($85) on 1/14/XX. Patient complained of pain in the ear and a sore throat. A diagnosis of otitis media and acute pharyngitis was determined. An injection of Cleocin was given ($30). Also an injection of Kenalog 40mg IM ($26). Symptoms first appeared 12/29/PY. A cash payment of $20 was made for this visit. The patient needs a receipt.

Item 20. ☐ **Y**ou check your IN box and find several charge slips. The following claim information was received from Dr. Ben Dover, Gastroenterologist. Enter these charges into the system.

CLAIM 10

Gene Poole received a comprehensive consultation of high complexity, performed at CHS Community Hospital ($310) on 1/8/XX. Patient was referred by Dr. Phil Goode. Inpatient problem focused, expanded exam was performed on 1/9/XX and on 1/10/XX ($75 each). Forty-five minute discharge was performed on 1/11/XX ($150). Diagnosis: Intestinal Obstruction, R/O Malignancy.

Item 21. ☐ **D**r. Dover asks you to estimate the patient's portion of the above charges and send the patient a bill. You call the insurance carrier and find out that Gene Poole has a $100 deductible and none of it has been paid. The insurance carrier pays 90%. Estimate the patient's portion of the above charges.

What are the total charges? _____

What is the estimated insurance payment? _____

What is the estimated patient portion? _____

Write a letter to the responsible party for the above patient requesting payment of the estimated portion of the patient's bill. Be sure to indicate that if the insurance carrier does not cover the entire billed amount there may be additional charges owed by the patient.

Item 22. ☐ **T**he following claim was received from Dr. Allotta Payne, OB-GYN. Enter these charges into the system.

CLAIM 11

Dee Pendent received a comprehensive, high complexity exam ($250), performed at CHS Community Hospital on 1/3/XX. Problem focused exams ($55 each) were performed on 1/5/XX, 1/7/XX, and 1/8/XX. Hospital discharge performed 1/9/XX ($115). Patient hospitalized 1/3/XX through 1/9/XX. Diagnosis: Condyloma, lower genital, Urosepsis, Acute UTI. A payment of $350 was made on the above charges by patient check #2135.

Item 23. ☐ **K**ent C. Theroad dances up to the window with a fun-loving smile. He takes one last spin and crashes into the wall. Righting himself, he sheepishly hands you a patient information sheet (Document 14) and a charge slip with the following information. Create a patient and family chart. Enter these charges into the system.

CLAIM 12

Dr. Sickman performed an intermediate ophthalmological exam on Kent C. Theroad in the office ($100) on 1/14/XX (date of first visit 9/17/PY). A blood specimen ($15) was taken. Diagnosis: Corneal Scars, Pterygium.

Item 24. ☐ **S**ue Pervisor, the office manager, has asked for a copy of your daily journal at the end of each day. A daily journal shows all transactions which occurred during a given day.

    ☞ Write up all transactions on a daily journal sheet.

     Print a day sheet. Use 01/14/XX as the date of the report. The report should include all entries.

Item 25. ☐ Print a transaction list. Use 01/14/XX as the date of the report. The report should include all entries.

    Check both of these reports. If there are any errors, correct them before proceeding.

Item 26. ☐ **P**rint or write up a deposit slip listing each check by number. Attach all checks and cash payments to the deposit slip.

Item 27. ☐ **R**econcile petty cash. Count all money remaining in petty cash and be sure you have the same amount left at the end of the day as you started with at the beginning. If not, determine exactly where the missing amount is.

Item 28. ☐ Print all the claims you have entered today. If you are using one-part forms, print two copies (see following exercise).

Item 29. ☐ **P**repare claims for mailing. Place one copy of the claim in the patient file. Place the second copy together with all claims for a single carrier. Print or write address labels and attach them to the claims.

Item 30. ☐ **I**s any additional information or confirmation needed regarding today's transactions? If so, what is it and how would you go about getting it?

_____

_____

_____

Item 31. ☐ **S**top and check that all assignments are correct before continuing on to the next date.

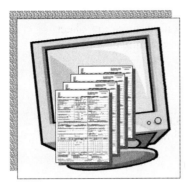

January 21, 20XX

Item 32. ☐ **T**oday's date is January 21, 20XX.

 Change the date to: January 21, 20XX.

Item 33. ☐ **C**ount petty cash. How much is in the cash envelope? _____

Item 34. ☐ **Y**ou check the fax machine and find a patient information sheet (Document 15). Something is wrong with the insurance information listed for one of the family members.

What is wrong and how would you fix it? _____

_____

Create a patient chart for these family members.

Item 35. ☐ **Y**ou receive a letter from Rover Insurers Inc. confirming that Codie Pendent has received pre-authorization for ten psychiatric treatments with Dr. Ben Looney, commencing on January 15, 20XX. The pre-authorization number is 1839A1B, authorized by D. Carrier. Dx: Adjustment Disorder.

    ☞ Complete an Authorized Treatment Form from the back of this book, and attach it to the patient's chart.

 Enter this information into the patient's record. If your computer system does not track authorized visits, use the Authorized Treatments Form from the back of this book.

Item 36. ☐ **D**r. Manny Kutz informs you that he has decided not to collect any remaining amounts due from Medicare patients. He will accept the amount that Medicare pays as payment in full. What do you do?

_____
_____
_____
_____
_____
_____
_____

Item 37. ☐ **Y**ou notice that some Medicare patients received services 11 months ago and Medicare was never billed. It appears that it was just an oversight. What do you do?

_____
_____
_____
_____
_____

Item 38. ☐ **A**s a medical biller, you should be familiar with at least some of the terms of the contracts for your patients. This allows you to inform the doctor and patient of any contract provisions which could provide greater insurance reimbursement. For example, some contracts pay 100% for pre-admission testing. Informing the doctor and patient of this allows them to make an informed decision regarding treatment.

At your request, Blue Corporation, Red Enterprises, and White Corporation have sent you copies of their contracts (Documents 16 – 18). Complete an insurance coverage sheet for each family. Blank insurance coverage sheets are in the Forms section in the back of this book. The completed insurance coverage sheets should be filed in the family's file, behind the patient information sheet.

When completing the insurance coverage sheets, list the name of the insured and their dependents across the bottom of the sheet. Use any previous claims and insurance payments to estimate the amount of deductible and coinsurance paid. This information should be considered estimated until confirmed by a phone call to the insurance carrier.

> ☞ Create an address list showing the name, phone number, and address of each of the insurance carriers. You may want to enter each company on a separate 3 X 5 card and place them in a card file box. This will allow you to create a new card and keep the file neat regardless of any changes for a company.

> 🖳 Be sure that the address and phone number information is correct, and complete in the Insurance Information screen on the computer. If incorrect or incomplete, update the information.

Item 39. ☐ **A** claim comes in from Dr. Phil Goode. Enter the charges into the system.

 CLAIM 13

Phillip D. Cupp received renal dialysis treatment at CHS outpatient department on 1/11/XX, and again on 1/14/XX ($115 each). Diagnosis: ESRD.

Item
40. ☐ **N**oah Account calls on the phone and says that he paid $30 in cash toward the bill on the day services were rendered, but it didn't show up on his statement. He says he did not bother to get a receipt. You check the patient's account and there is no record of the payment. What do you do?

_____

_____

_____

_____

_____

_____

Item
41. ☐ **Y**ou cover for Dr. Yu B. Sickman's receptionist while she goes to the bank and to lunch. The clipboards are already made up with blank patient information sheets and medical histories for the patient to complete. Neva Tu Early enters the office with her son, Barry Tired, who has not been feeling well. "He seems to be spending all his time in bed and never feels like getting up," she complains. She completes the patient information sheet for her family (Document 19). When finished, Barry is seen by Dr. Sickman. Mrs. Early is unsure whose insurance pays first for Barry. "He's the son of my first husband and I, and he has insurance through both of us, though he lives with my new husband and me. I've filled out the chart as much as I can."
     Determine the correct order of insurance, then make up a family and patient chart.

What questions should be asked of Mrs. Early to help you determine the correct order of insurance carriers? _____

_____

_____

Why is it important for you to know where Barry lives to determine the correct order of insurance carriers?

_____

_____

 Enter the patient information into the computer.

Item
42. ☐ **C**ab N. Fever enters the office with his children, Scarlet and Ty Phoid. The family had been hiking in the woods this morning on Mount Mountain. Ty has asthma and had an asthmatic attack. He is having dyspnea, though not severe. His father would like him checked out. Mr. Fever fills out a patient information sheet (Document 20). He is unsure of the correct payment order for the insurances which cover his children. Determine the correct order of insurance, then create family and patient charts. Also be sure to add the diagnosis of asthma to Ty's patient information sheet if it was not listed by his father.

 Enter the patient information into the computer.

Item 43. ☐ **M**rs. Valasquez comes in carrying her five-year-old daughter, Veronica. She states that she needs to see the doctor. They do not have an appointment, but Mrs. Valasquez says that Veronica is running a bit of a fever and does not feel well. She thinks Veronica may have the mumps. The doctor is running a little late and the waiting room is full of patients who do have appointments. What do you do?

_____

_____

_____

_____

_____

_____

_____

Item 44. ☐ **M**rs. Early comes out of the treatment room with Barry. She hands you the following list of charges for Barry's visit:

CLAIM 14

Established office visit, high complexity	$190
CBC	$ 30
HIV 1 & 2 test	$ 30
Hepatitis B test	$ 30
T cell count	$ 30

Diagnosis: Malaise, Muscular Weakness, R/O HIV, R/O Hepatitis.
Mrs. Early pays $25 in cash.

Enter the charges into the system.

Item 45. ☐ **D**. Jobb Dunnitt steps out of the treatment room with his daughter V. Iris Dunnitt. He hands you a charge slip showing the following charges. Enter the charges into the system.

CLAIM 15

Dr. Sickman performed a problem focused office visit ($55) on V. Iris. Diagnosis: Rhinovirus.

Mr. Dunnitt asks how much the patient's portion for the visit will be. You contact his insurance carrier and find that V. Iris has not yet paid any of her deductible. Using the information contained on the patient insurance coverage sheet, determine how much the deductible and estimated patient's portion of the bill will be.

What are the total charges?_____

What is the estimated insurance payment?_____

What is the estimated patient portion? _____

Mr. Dunnitt writes a check (#1805 in the Windows Payment Section) for the above amount and asks for a receipt. Fill in the amount on the patient's check.

☞ Write out a receipt for Mr. Dunnitt.

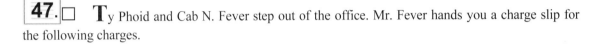 Return to the transaction screen, enter the payment, and print him a walkout receipt.

 46. ☐ **A** man walks in with a skinned knee, compound fracture of the right arm, and blood streaming from a gash on his head. He says, "Hello, I'm Mr. Tern Wong. I was riding my bike when I lost control and hit a tree. I'm not a regular patient, but I think I need to see the doctor." The doctor is in a confidential meeting with a patient and has told you not to disturb him for any reason. What do you do?

_____

_____

_____

_____

_____

47. ☐ **T**y Phoid and Cab N. Fever step out of the office. Mr. Fever hands you a charge slip for the following charges.

 CLAIM 16
Ty received an office visit, low complexity ($150). Diagnosis: Asthma, Dyspnea.

48. ☐ **Y**ou return to your own desk in the billing office. Sue Pervisor says that they have received updated UCR information on some of the procedures and have decided to revise the costs for a few of them (Document 21).

☞ Store this information with (Document 4) and keep them in an accessible place.

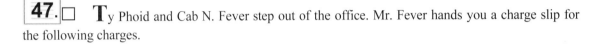 Using the Procedure Code Information screen, update the charges in the computer.

49. ☐ **Y**ou find claim information on the following patient visits in your IN box. Enter these charges into the system.

CLAIM 17
Codie Pendent received individual psychotherapy performed by Dr. Ben Looney, Psychiatrist, in the office on 1/17/XX ($160). Individual psychological testing was administered for five hours on 1/17/XX ($575). Diagnosis: Adjustment Disorder.

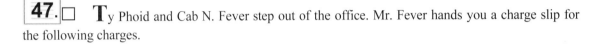 Remember to fill out the authorized visits chart for any psychiatric treatments received by Codie Pendent.

CLAIM 18
Jeanette Akenja-Nearing received a routine pregnancy exam ($55), ultrasound ($190), and urinalysis ($30) in the office on 1/13/XX, along with a Hepatitis B test ($30). Services were performed by Dr. Allotta Payne, OB-GYN. Patient is due 2/27/XX.

Item
50. ☐   **M**aria Gonzalez, a new mother, calls up and says her three-month-old daughter has had a bad case of diarrhea and has been spitting up a bit for the past two days. The child does not seem to be running a fever, but she has been fussy and does not want to take her bottle. Maria wants to know if she should bring the child in to see Dr. Sickman, and if so, when is there an appointment open? The next available appointment is in ten days. What do you say?

_____

_____

_____

_____

_____

_____

_____

_____

Item
51. ☐   **M**r. Shay Kee Hart toddles up to the window with a new patient information sheet (Document 22). He has just been seen by Dr. Yu B. Sickman and the following services were rendered. Make up a patient chart and enter the following charges into the system.

CLAIM 19
Office visit, established, high complexity ($190), Urinalysis ($30). Diagnosis: Lou Gehrig's Disease.

When you finish with the claim form, Mr. Hart announces, "I would like to pay for the estimated patient portion of the visit at this time, including my yearly deductible. Here's my check (#1796 from the Window Payments section). You can fill in the amount for me. I would also like something showing me how you came up with my amount and a receipt for it."

Create the information Mr. Hart wants, and then complete the check and process the payment.

Item
52. ☐   **M**r. Hart is still at the window when you finish. When you ask if there is something else you can do for him, he replies, "You can send the claim to Medicare, but I need to get a second copy of the claim form to send to my other insurance carrier. Could you please print out a second claim? My wife just got out of the hospital from a heart attack and the second insurance carrier has had problems in the past. I want to send this one in myself, certified mail, so they can't say they didn't get it." What do you say or do?

_____

_____

_____

_____

_____

Item
53. ☐   **T**ake a moment to make sure all patient charts are up to date and are placed neatly in alphabetical order.

Item 54. ☐ **Y**ou check your IN box and find several charge slips. The following claim information was received from Dr. Yu B. Sickman. Enter these charges into the system.

CLAIM 20

Ron E. Knose received an expanded exam with low complexity in the office on 1/20/XX ($85). His symptoms first appeared on 12/29/PY. He had previously seen Dr. Goode, but his symptoms have not cleared. An injection of penicillin was given ($25). Also a throat culture was done ($20) and a Urine dip ($30). Diagnosis: Upper Respiratory Infection.

CLAIM 21

While in the morgue of CHS Community Hospital, a lab specimen was collected from Mort Allity and sent to the lab for performance of a Hemogram with platelet and differential ($11) and CPK ($56) on 1/17/XX. Also on 1/17/XX, an amylase test ($19) and comprehensive metabolic panel was ordered ($130), and on 1/18/XX, LDH, lactic acid ($16). All tests were ordered by Dr. Yu B. Sickman, who interpreted the results. Diagnosis: Unattended Death. Body arrived 1/17/XX and was released 1/21/XX.

CLAIM 22

Carla Poole was brought into the office on 1/14/XX with a laceration of the left index finger. Mr. Poole stated that Carla's finger was run over by a skate on 1/8/XX. Finger appears to be infected. An expanded visit of low complexity was performed ($85). An x-ray of the finger was done ($40). A sterile tray was used ($50) to prep and wrap the finger.

CLAIM 23

On 1/6/XX a car was erratically driven into the emergency entrance of CHS Hospital, heedless of the pedestrians exiting the building. Brooke N. Hart stumbled out and staggered into the ER complaining of severe chest pain. Dr. Sickman immediately performed a high complexity visit ($195) and an EKG with report ($40). After letting her rest for a bit, Dr. Sickman made her perform a treadmill test with report ($170). Brooke also received a CBC with platelet count ($50), thyroid hormone test ($50), and hepatic panel ($45). Diagnosis: Chest Pain, Cardiac Arrhythmia, Myocardial Infarction.

CLAIM 24

Dr. Sickman decided that Brooke N. Hart's condition required hospitalization. He performed a comprehensive, high complexity hospital admit ($250) on 1/7/XX. Mrs. Hart was prepared for surgery on 1/8/XX with the following tests performed: blood typing and RH ($35), ABG, pH only ($75). A combined right heart catheterization and transseptal left heart catheterization through intact septum ($3,650) was performed. Dr. Sickman performed expanded follow-up visits on 1/9/XX, 1/10/XX, 1/11/XX, and 1/12/XX ($75 each). A discharge visit was performed 1/13/XX ($115). Diagnosis: A/P CABG/Coronary Artery Bypass, ASHD/CAD. Hospitalized: 1/7/XX through 1/13/XX.

CLAIM 25

Hick Cupp received a computerized visual field, extended test ($110) on 1/17/XX. A new patient comprehensive eye exam with no refraction ($205) was performed on 1/18/XX. Diagnosis: Cataract Nuclearsclerotic.

Item 55. ☐ The auditors have just finished checking last year's accounts. They needed more information for why adjustments were made in order for them to be allowed. The entire office spent numerous hours looking up the information in the patient records. In order to prevent this from happening again, Sue Pervisor has created additional procedure codes which further clarify why adjustments were made (Document 23).

> ☞ Keep this list handy for use with all future adjustment entries.

> 🖳 Enter these codes and descriptions into the Procedure Code Information screen. Be sure that when you abbreviate the description, all pertinent information is included.

Item 56. ☐ Now write a memo to all doctors and staff to inform them of the new codes and let them know that anyone making an adjustment needs to clarify the reason for the adjustment. The memo should also mention to those who put information into the computerized system that they should start using the new codes immediately and that whenever any of the codes are used, any additional pertinent information should be included in the diagnosis column (i.e., if a code was entered in error, list both the old code and the new code in the diagnosis space).

Item 57. ☐ Dr. Sickman's receptionist has set up a number of appointments in Dr. Sickman's calendar (Document 10). She asks you to add these to the computer, and also schedule the following appointments in the doctor's appointment calendar.

Pat Prescott would like an appointment on 1/22/XX at 3 p.m. for 30 minutes.

Using the information contained in Document 4, determine the best time for the following two appointments:
Wayne Wu would like an appointment on 1/22/XX for an established, expanded, low complexity exam. Lee Li would like an appointment on 1/22/XX for a new patient high complexity exam.

Item 58. ☐ Dr. Will Kutteroff calls and asks you to schedule inpatient surgery for Rhea Ality for excision of a pilonidal cyst on 2/1/XX from 2:30 p.m. to 4 p.m. at CHS Community Hospital. Place the information for the surgery in the doctor's appointment schedule. Is there anything you should bring to the doctor's attention?

_____

_____

_____

_____

Item 59. ☐ When you return from lunch you find some mail on your desk. You open the mail to find a new patient information sheet (Document 24). Make up patient and family charts.

> 🖳 Enter the data into the computer.

Item 60. ☐ Mr. Eaton Wright, an elderly patient, steps up to the window and says he has just been diagnosed with diabetes. He seems stunned. He asks if you can tell him any more about the disease. He is asking you because he does not want to take up any more of the doctor's time. What do you do?

Item
61. ☐ **T**he doctor has put Mr. Wright on a special diet. He will also need daily insulin injections. You know the patient has had difficulty paying his bills and you are not sure if he will be able to afford the diet, insulin, or other paraphernalia necessary to monitor his condition. What do you do?

Item
62. ☐ **M**r. Al Weighs Knose calls up and says he needs to make another payment on his bill. He asks you to fax him a copy of his latest statement to fax number 555-0192. What do you do?

Item
63. ☐ **M**r. Juan Mai Moni, a new patient, steps up to the window with his patient information sheet. He refuses to sign the authorization to release information because the wording of the statement also includes assignment of benefits. The patient does not have a problem with you releasing the information, but he wants the insurance company to pay him rather than paying the doctor. What do you do?

Item
64. ☐ **S**herry Attricks steps up to the window with a charge slip. Enter these charges into the system.

 CLAIM 26

Sherry Attricks had the following tests performed in the office on 1/21/XX by Dr. Yu B. Sickman. Basic Metabolic Panel ($80), sodium ($21), potassium ($21), cholesterol ($25), and calcium ($20). Diagnosis: Venous Insufficiency, Varicose Veins. The patient pays $45 for this visit by check #1932. Ms. Attricks would like a receipt.

Item
65. ☐ **P**rint or write up a day sheet or daily journal.

Item
66. ☐ **P**rint or write up a deposit slip for all monies received. Attach all checks and cash payments to it.

Item 67. ☐ **R**econcile petty cash. Count all money remaining in petty cash and be sure you have the same amount left at the end of the day as you started with at the beginning. If not, determine exactly where the missing amount is.

Item 68. ☐ Print all the claims you have entered today. If you are using one-part forms, print two copies (see following exercise).

Item 69. ☐ **P**repare claims for mailing. Place one copy of the claim in the patient file. Place the second copy together with all claims for a single carrier. Print or write address labels and attach them to the claims.

Item 70. ☐ **A**n insurance carrier calls and says they have overpaid a claim. They would like you to send them a check for $135, the amount of the overpayment. What do you do?

_____

_____

_____

_____

_____

Item 71. ☐ **D**r. Phil Goode would like a copy of his appointment schedule for tomorrow.

☞ Make a copy of Dr. Goode's appointments.

 Print Dr. Goode's appointments off the computer.

Item 72. ☐ **D**r. Sickman would like you to prepare charge slips for the patients he will see tomorrow.

☞ Using the charge slips in the back of this text and the appointment calendar (Document 10), make up one for each patient the doctor will be seeing tomorrow.

 Print charge slips from the computer.

Item 73. ☐ **I**s any additional information or confirmation needed for today's transactions? If so, what?

_____

_____

_____

_____

_____

Item 74. ☐ **S**top and check that all assignments are correct before continuing on to the next date.

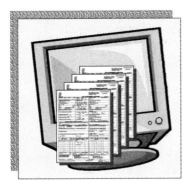

February 4, 20XX

Item 75. ☐ **T**oday's date is February 4, 20XX.

 Change the date to: February 4, 20XX.

Item 76. ☐ **C**ount petty cash. How much is in the cash envelope? _____

Item 77. ☐ **D**r. Goode's receptionist is having car trouble and you are asked to cover the front desk for her until she gets in. Just as you sit down, a woman comes in to the office with a young child who appears to be in pain. Neither the woman nor the child speaks English, and no one seems to understand the language they are speaking. The woman is getting more and more frantic. What do you do?

_____

_____

_____

_____

Item 78. ☐ **M**rs. Harenstein brings her teenage daughter Hanna in. Hanna has slashed her own wrists, but the wounds are little more than scratches. Mrs. Harenstein does not seem to be taking the incident seriously and says, "Oh, it's just her way of getting attention." What do you do?

_____

_____

_____

_____

Item 79. ☐ **M**rs. Begay comes in and states that she is moving out of town this afternoon and therefore she will be transferring her daughter's care to another physician. Her daughter has a heart condition and needs constant care and monitoring. She is in a hurry and would like her daughter's chart immediately. What do you do?

_____

_____

_____

_____

_____

_____

_____

_____

Item 80. ☐ **W**hen you arrive back at your desk, there are several pieces of mail waiting for you. Included in the mail is a detailing of charges paid by Winter Insurance, one of the insurance carriers (Document 25). Credit the appropriate amounts to the correct accounts, then do any balance billing to either the patient or an additional insurance carrier. When billing a secondary insurance payor, be sure to attach a copy of the EOB. Data for other patients should be redacted (blacked out). A secondary copy of the EOB need not be attached when you are balance billing the patient. The insurance carrier should have already sent them a copy of the EOB.

☞ Do not forget to update the patient ledger cards to reflect the payments.

Item 81. ☐ **T**hree envelopes contain patient checks (Document 26). Credit these payments to the proper accounts.

Item 82. ☐ **D**. Jobb Dunnitt steps up to the window with a charge slip. Enter these charges into the system.

CLAIM 27

Candy Dunnitt was seen by Dr. Sickman today for Diabetes Mellitus. An expanded exam with history was performed ($85) in the office. A routine blood glucose strip was done ($40) to check the blood sugar.

Item 83. ☐ **A**lso included in the mail is a detailing of charges paid by Rover Insurers, Inc. and Ball Insurance Carriers, two of the insurance carriers (Documents 27 and 28). Credit the appropriate amounts to the correct accounts, then do any balance billing to either the patient or an additional insurance carrier. When billing a secondary insurance payor, be sure to attach a copy of the EOB. Data for other patients should be redacted (blacked-out). A copy of the EOB need not be attached when you are balance billing the patient. The insurance carrier should have already sent them a copy of the EOB.

Item 84. ☐ **T**he patient statement for the Goway family is returned in the mail marked "Addressee has moved." There is a balance due of $545 on the account. You call the phone number listed in the patient's chart and find that the number has been disconnected. What do you do?

_____

_____

_____

_____

_____

_____

85. ☐ **Y**ou check your IN box and find several charge slips. The following claim information was received from Dr. Phil Goode. Enter these charges into the system.

  CLAIM 28

Phillip D. Cupp received renal dialysis treatment at CHS outpatient department on 1/17/XX, 1/22/XX, 1/25/XX, and 1/27/XX ($115 each). Services were performed by Dr. Phil Goode. Diagnosis: ESRD.

86. ☐ **T**he following claim information was received from Dr. Ben Dover, Gastroenterologist. Enter these charges into the system.

  CLAIM 29

Petey Attricks received a hospital admit of moderate complexity performed on 1/14/XX ($180). On 1/15/XX, Dr. Dover performed a cholecystectomy with exploration of common duct ($1,720). Follow-up hospital visits were performed on 1/16/XX, 1/17/XX ($95 each), and a discharge was performed on 1/18/XX ($150). Diagnosis: Calculus Cholecystitis. Patient hospitalized 1/14/XX through 1/18/XX at CHS Community Hospital.

CLAIM 30

Office surgery was performed by Dr. Ben Dover on Andy Pendent for a diagnosis of hemorrhoids. An anoscopy ($130) was performed on 1/17/XX. A hemorrhoidectomy, external, complete ($550) was also performed on 1/17/XX. Proctosigmoidoscopy ($100) and removal of polyp ($75) were performed on 1/18/XX. Mr. Pendent made a cash payment of $50 on 1/18/XX.

87. ☐ **D**r. Dover asks you to estimate the patient's portion of the above charges and send the patient a bill.

For Petey Attricks:

You call the insurance carrier and find out that he has not satisfied any of his deductible. However, you had previously sent in a bill for this patient which has probably not been paid by the insurance carrier yet. Use the insurance coverage sheet to determine his deductible. Estimate the patient's portion of the above charges.

What are the total charges? _____

What is the estimated insurance payment? _____

What is the estimated patient portion? _____

For Andy Pendent:

You call the insurance carrier and find out that Mr. Pendent has not satisfied any of his deductible. Use the insurance coverage sheet to determine his deductible. Estimate the patient's portion of the above charges.

What are the total charges?_____

What is the estimated insurance payment?_____

What is the estimated patient portion?_____

How much was paid by the patient?_____

How much does the patient still owe?_____

Write a letter to the responsible party for each of the above patients requesting payment of the estimated portion of the patient's bill. Be sure to indicate that if the insurance carrier does not cover the entire billed amount there may be additional charges owed by the patient.

 88. ☐ **D**r. Goode asks you to send a letter to Mr. Noah Listen, a patient, stating that he will no longer agree to see him because he does not follow the medical advice the doctor gives. What do you do? If you would write the letter, draft it on the stationery in the back of this book.

_____

_____

_____

_____

_____

_____

 89. ☐ **T**he following claim information was received from Dr. Ben Looney, Psychiatrist. Enter these charges into the system.

 CLAIM 31

Codie Pendent received individual psychotherapy in the office on 1/23/XX and 1/30/XX ($160 each). Diagnosis: Adjustment Disorder. Date First Seen: 1/14/XX.

☞ Remember to fill out the authorized visits chart for any psychiatric treatments received by Codie Pendent.

90. ☐ **T**he following claim information was received from Dr. Yu B. Sickman. Enter these charges into the system.

CLAIM 32

D. Jobb Dunnitt came into the ER complaining of difficulty breathing. A problem focused exam with straightforward decision making was performed in the emergency room ($120) on 1/23/XX. Dr. Sickman ordered a complete blood count with manual differential ($25) and a CO_2 response curve ($80). Because the patient was diagnosed with chronic bronchitis, a chest x-ray with two views was performed ($60). The patient was also diagnosed with Asbestosis. The first visit pertaining to this illness was on 1/9/XX. A payment of $60 was made for this visit by patient check #1809. The patient requests a receipt.

Remember to add the diagnoses of Chronic Bronchitis and Asbestosis to the patient information sheet if they are not already indicated.

CLAIM 33

Dee Pendent was brought into the office on 1/22/XX by her mother. Mrs. Pendent stated that Dee tripped at home and hit her head on the cement driveway. She was treated for a bloody nose and complained of headache and neck stiffness. A detailed exam of moderate complexity was performed ($130). A complete x-ray of the skull was taken ($85). Also a complete x-ray of the cervical spine was done ($100).

CLAIM 34

D. Jobb Dunnitt was seen by the physician's assistant in the office on 2/1/XX for an established patient office visit ($40). Diagnosis: Bronchitis.

CLAIM 35

Hugh Waite limped into the office on 1/11/XX complaining of an ingrown toenail of the left hallux. Dr. Sickman performed a left border matrixectomy ($200) and a right border matrixectomy ($200) in the office. A $400 payment was made by patient (check #1298).

Item 91. ☐ **S**hay Kee Hart staggers up to the window with the following charge slip. Enter these charges into the system.

CLAIM 36

Shay Kee Hart received physical therapy from Dr. Sickman for 45 minutes ($135), a whirlpool treatment ($25), and non-direct traction ($25) on 01/28/XX. The same treatments were repeated on 2/4/XX. On 2/4/XX he was also given 2.5 mg. of Methotrexate (orally) ($30). Diagnosis: Amyotrophic Lateral Sclerosis. Mr. Hart asks you to estimate his portion of the charges.

What are the total charges?_____

What is the estimated insurance payment?_____

What is the estimated patient portion?_____

Mr. Hart writes check #1835 to cover his portion of the charges. Fill in the amount of the check.

Item 92. ☐ **R**eturn to entering Dr. Sickman's charges.

CLAIM 37

A comprehensive exam with history was performed on Cass N. O'Gen in the office ($190) on 1/29/XX. Because of a history of fibrocystic breast disease, a bilateral mammography was performed ($82). Patient complained of pelvic pain, requiring a complete pelvic ultrasound ($100). Upper respiratory infection was also diagnosed and three views of the paranasal sinuses were taken ($50). A blood specimen was collected for further testing

($15). Patient was referred to Dr. Allotta Payne, OB-GYN. A payment of $125 was made on the above charges by patient (check #2938). Patient requests a receipt.

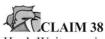**CLAIM 38**

Hugh Waite received an expanded office visit of low complexity ($85) on 1/27/XX. Biopsy of one skin lesion ($130) was also performed, and an additional four lesions were biopsied ($45 each). On 1/28/XX a matrixectomy of the R Hallux by laser ($250) and matrixectomy of the L Hallux ($250) were performed. Sterile surgical tray ($100), surgical drape ($50), laser usage fee ($100), and operating room fee ($200) were also billed. Diagnosis: Infected Mycotic Nails, both great toes, Onychomycosis, painful Keratoderma, first digit bilateral.

Item 93. ☐ **D**r. Allotta Payne calls and asks you to schedule Cass N. O'Gen for ovarian mass surgery. She states that she can perform surgery on either February 12th or February 19th. Dr. Payne does not care which day the surgery is scheduled for. Upon contacting the patient's mother, Pat N. O'Gen, she asks what day you think her daughter should have the surgery. What is your response?

_____
_____
_____
_____
_____
_____

Ms. O'Gen says that she would rather have the surgery scheduled for February 12th. Schedule the surgery in Dr. Payne's appointment calendar. The surgery will start at 4 p.m. and will last approximately three and a half hours.

Item 94. ☐ **A** sealed letter is dropped on your desk from Dr. Goode. You open it to find a letter that had been addressed to Dr. Phil Goode. A copy is now forwarded to you with some personal information blacked out (Document 29). Change the information in the patient's record. If necessary, complete a new patient information sheet.

 Change the data in the patient information screen.

Item 95. ☐ **D**r. Goode's receptionist calls from her office and says that Al Weighs Knose is bringing his son Beane in to be looked at. She believes this family has unpaid bills from previous visits and would like to have a copy of the family's statements.

☞ Make a copy of the statements for all family members or write the data from all family members on a single patient ledger card.

 Print out the statements for all family members.

Additionally, the current visit seems to require a low complexity office visit. Let her know what the charge is for this service so she can collect what she can from Mr. Knose.

How much does this family still owe for previous visits? _____

How much is the standard charge for a low complexity office visit?_____

What is the total of these two amounts?_____

Does the patient have any insurance which may cover a portion of the charges? If so, approximately how much will the insurance cover?_____

 96. ☐ **M**r. Fraide sends in a revised patient information sheet (Document 30) with a letter stating that his wife has begun working full-time and now there is insurance for the family under both his policy and his wife's policy. Determine which policy will be primary and which secondary for each person and write it on the patient information sheet. Update the patients' charts by replacing the old patient information sheet with the new one.

 Enter the corrected data into the computer.

97. ☐ **S**ue Pervisor asks you to let all patients know about a health fair that is coming up on March 12 between 8 a.m. and 6 p.m. at the Community Center, 10911 Capshaw Drive, Colton, CO. For more information, patients can call the office. Compose a memo to be added into the envelope containing the patient statements. Use the stationery at the back of this book.

98. ☐ **D**r. Goode's receptionist steps in and hands you a check from Al Weighs Knose in the amount of $75.00 (check #2245). She also hands you a charge slip for services rendered to Ron E. Knose. Enter the charges into the system.

CLAIM 39

Ron E. Knose received a low complexity office visit ($85) and a urinalysis ($30). Diagnosis: Flu. Enter the charges into the system and apply the $75 payment to these current charges.

How much is now owed by the members of the Knose family?_____

99. ☐ **A** few charge slips are dropped in your IN box. The following claim information was received from Dr. Allotta Payne, OB-GYN. Enter the charges into the system.

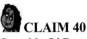 **CLAIM 40**

Cass N. O'Gen received an initial consultation and comprehensive, moderate complexity visit performed at CHS Community Hospital outpatient department ($275) on 2/1/XX. Patient was referred by Dr. Yu B. Sickman. Diagnosis: Left Ovarian Mass, Pelvis Adhesions.

100. ☐ **T**he following claim information was received from Dr. Will Kutteroff, Surgeon. Enter the charges into the system.

CLAIM 41

On 2/1/XX, Dr. Kutteroff performed an excision of pilonidal cyst ($380) at the outpatient department of CHS Community Hospital on Rhea Allity.

CLAIM 42

P'Lisa Waite received a capsulotomy, extensive, including posterior ($1,950) at CHS Community Hospital on 1/8/XX. Diagnosis: Clubfoot. Hospitalized: 1/8/XX to 1/11/XX.

Item 101. ☐ **A**n insurance carrier has not acknowledged a claim, so you call to find out what is happening. Once before the claims examiner had said they never received the claim. They again say they never received it. What do you do?

_____

_____

_____

_____

_____

_____

Item 102. ☐ **D**r. Anne S. Thesia, Anesthesiologist, provided anesthesia during the following operations. Dr. Thesia is a new provider and will need to be added into the system.

☞ Write in the data for Dr. Thesia on the provider information sheet.

🖳 Add Dr. Thesia to the Provider Information screen.

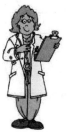

Provider:	Anne S. Thesia, M.D. Anesthesiologist
Address:	1357 Castle Blvd, Ste. 511, Colter, CO 81222
Phone:	(970) 555-3482
License #:	AST47028
EIN:	40-3445555
MCR UPIN:	AST098

Provider Accepts Medicare Assignment

Item 103. ☐ **N**ow enter the charges provided by Dr. Thesia into the system.

CLAIM 43

Cholecystectomy with exploration of common duct ($2,550) performed on Petey Attricks on 1/15/XX. Dx: Calculus Cholecystitis. Total anesthesia time: 08:20 - 11:35.

CLAIM 44

A complete stripping of long, saphenous vein right leg ($1,000) performed on Sherry Attricks on 2/1/XX. Dx: Venous Insufficiency, Varicose Veins. Total anesthesia time: 9:55 - 11:30.

CLAIM 45

Excision of pilonidal cyst ($1,300) performed on Rhea Allity at the outpatient department of CHS Community Hospital on 2/1/XX. Total anesthesia time: 14:30 - 15:35.

CLAIM 46

P'Lisa Waite received a capsulotomy, extensive, including posterior ($2,851) at CHS Community Hospital on 1/8/XX. Dx: Clubfoot. Hospitalized: 1/8/XX to 1/11/XX.

Item 104. ☐ **M**s. Penny Less, a patient, has a condition which the insurance company has determined to be a pre-existing condition. She is covered by the White Corporation contract. You know Ms. Less has financial difficulties and you are concerned this may affect her seeking treatment. What do you do?

_____
_____
_____
_____
_____
_____

Item 105. ☐ **T**he phone rings. Codie Pendent is on the line. "Hello, I'm sorry to bother you, but I'm seeing Dr. Looney. My insurance carrier allowed only a certain number of visits, but I forgot how many. Can you tell me how many they authorized and how many visits are left that they will cover?" What do you say?

_____
_____
_____
_____
_____

Item 106. ☐ **Y**ou receive a claim back from Rover Insurers, saying that Don T. Cover, a patient for whom you sent in a claim, is not covered by them. What do you do?

_____
_____
_____
_____

Item 107. ☐ **P**rint or write up a day sheet or daily journal.

Item 108. ☐ **P**rint or write up a deposit slip for all monies received. Attach all checks and cash payments to it.

Item 109. ☐ **R**econcile petty cash. Count all money remaining in petty cash and be sure you have the same amount left at the end of the day as you started with at the beginning. If not, determine exactly where the missing amount is.

Item 110. ☐ Print all the claims you have entered today. If you are using one-part forms, print two copies (see following exercise).

Item 111. ☐ **P**repare claims for mailing. Place one copy of the claim in the patient file. Place the second copy together with all claims for a single carrier. Print or write address labels and attach them to the claims.

Item 112. ☐ **P**atient statements for the month of January need to be mailed out.

☞ Make sure that all patient ledgers have been updated and are showing correct balances due. Make a copy of those that have balances of more than $1.

 Print patient statements for all patients with balances over $1.

Item 113. ☐ **I**s any additional information or confirmation needed for today's transactions? If so, what?

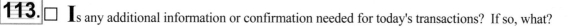

_____

_____

_____

_____

_____

Item 114. ☐ **S**top and check that all assignments are correct before continuing on to the next date.

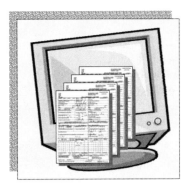

March 4, 20XX

Item
115. ☐ **T**oday's date is March 4, 20XX.

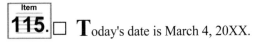 Change the date to: March 4, 20XX.

Item
116. ☐ **C**ount petty cash. How much is in the cash envelope? ....

Item
117. ☐ **S**ue Pervisor announces that CHS Community Hospital has had a fire and lost much of their computer data. Itemized bills for many accounts were printed, but a UB-92 was not completed for these patients. They ask for your assistance. Please complete UB-92s for the patient bills shown in Documents 31 – 35. These claims are for hospital charges, so they will not be entered into your system. Because of this, and because many medical billing programs do not generate hospital billing forms, the UB-92s will need to be completed manually.

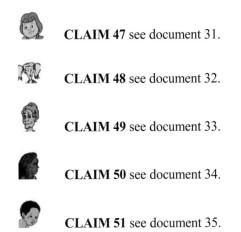

                     CLAIM 47 see document 31.

                     CLAIM 48 see document 32.

                     CLAIM 49 see document 33.

                     CLAIM 50 see document 34.

                     CLAIM 51 see document 35.

Item

118. ☐ **T**he following claim information was received from Dr. Allotta Payne, OB-GYN. Enter the charges into the system.

CLAIM 52

According to the patient record of Jeanette Akenja-Nearing, a detailed office visit ($70) was performed on 7/2/PY. Follow-up office visits were performed on 8/16/PY, 9/21/PY, 10/16/PY, and 11/21/PY, all for $50 each. A UA dip with micro ($10) was performed on 11/21/PY. Jeanette vaginally delivered a baby boy on 2/25/XX ($2,500), and promptly named him Wade N. Poole. None of these charges were previously billed. Diagnosis: Pregnancy. Patient hospitalized 2/25/XX to 2/26/XX. A payment of $1,500 was made by patient check #1815.

CLAIM 53

Cass N. O'Gen was scheduled for surgery at CHS Community Hospital on 2/12/XX. Dr. Allotta Payne, OB-GYN, performed a hysterectomy ($1,250), oophorectomy ($750), laparoscopy with lysis of adhesions ($785), dilation of vagina under anesthesia ($175), and D&C ($275). Diagnosis: Left Ovarian Mass, Pelvic Adhesions, Severe Recto-Cystocele. First seen: 1/29/XX.

Item

119. ☐ **D**r. Anne S. Thesia sends you a note indicating that the anesthesia time on P'Lisa Waite's surgery was 2 hours and 35 min (claim 46). Finish billing this claim. If you previously sent in P'Lisa Waite's claim without anesthesia time, complete another CMS-1500 and write a cover letter saying that this claim replaces the old one and why.

If you previously entered P'Lisa Waite's claim, complete the claim information.

Item

120. ☐ **C**hecks from three insurance carriers are received in the mail (Documents 36 – 38). Credit the appropriate amounts to the correct accounts, then do any balance billing to either the patient or an additional insurance carrier. When billing a secondary insurance payor, be sure to attach a copy of the EOB. Data for other patients should be redacted. A copy of the EOB need not be attached when you are balance billing the patient. The insurance carrier should have already sent them a copy of the EOB.

Item

121. ☐ **Y**ou receive an insurance payment for a number of claims, one of which appears to be incorrect. In double-checking the patient's account you discover that you coded a procedure incorrectly and have been reimbursed for the wrong amount. The amount is less than the doctor billed, but probably more than would be paid if the claim had been coded correctly. What do you do?

_____

_____

_____

_____

_____

_____

Item 122. ☐ Sue Pervisor asks you for an insurance aging report. Create or print out the report. This will be used to contact insurance carriers who have not made payment on claims submitted over 30 days or more. It should include all insurance carriers.

> ☞ Using the Insurance Aging Report form in the back of this book, create an Insurance Aging Report.

> Print out an Insurance Aging Report.

Item 123. ☐ Checks come in from five patients (Document 39). Credit the proper accounts, then do any balance billing to either the patient or an additional insurance carrier. When billing a secondary insurance payor, be sure to attach a copy of the EOB. Data for other patients should be redacted. A copy of the EOB need not be attached when you are balance billing the patient. The insurance carrier should have already sent them a copy of the EOB.

Item 124. ☐ You forgot to enter the words "Signature on File" in the Assignment of Benefits box on Minnie Mumwage's claim. You call the insurance carrier and they state that since the box was not signed, they sent payment to the patient. The claim was for $575 and they made a payment for $321.77. What do you do?

_____

_____

_____

_____

_____

_____

Item 125. ☐ You call Minnie Mumwage and she tearfully says she does not have the money to cover the above charges. She spent it for food and rent. "Besides," she says belligerently, "it was your mistake. You should pay for it." What do you do?

_____

_____

_____

_____

Item 126. ☐ ER reports shown in Document 40 are dropped in your IN box detailing an accident involving the Theroad Family. Bill for the services.

 CLAIM 54 see document 40.

 CLAIM 55 see document 40.

CLAIM 56 see document 40.

 CLAIM 57 see document 40.

In order to provide the best benefit for the family, which of the claims should be submitted first and why?

_____

_____

_____

_____

_____

_____

Item 127. ☐ **C**harge slips showing ER services for two other patients are also in your box. Bill for these services.

CLAIM 58

A crying Dee Pendent was brought into the emergency room of CHS Community Hospital on 2/3/XX by her mother. Mrs. Pendent stated that the patient fell from a horse today. Open treatment of distal radial fx ($450) was performed by Dr. Noah Pulse.

CLAIM 59

Late in the evening on 3/1/XX, Jeanette Akenja-Nearing frantically rushed into the ER with her newborn son, Wade N. Poole, in her arms. Her husband, Gene Poole, was at her side, with one arm around his wife and the other around their daughter Carla. "We put him to bed at 8 o'clock, but when we checked on him about an hour later, he wasn't breathing," Jeanette cried out.

"We did CPR and he seems to be breathing better now," Gene added. "Please help us." Dr. Noah Pulse immediately took the child and performed a comprehensive, high complexity exam ($240). Wade was admitted for observation. Diagnosis: Apnea.

Item 128. ☐ **A**l Weighs Knose steps up to the window with his nose in the air and a charge slip in his hand. Enter the charges into the system.

CLAIM 60

Beane Andy Knose was brought into Dr. Goode's office today complaining of "something in my nose." Upon examination, a kidney bean was removed from the right nostril ($360). During examination the doctor also noted excessive ear wax which resulted in ear lavage ($80).

Al Weighs Knose writes a check (#2261) for $50 for these services. In the "For:" section of the check is written "Payment in full for all medical services." How much is owed on this account?_____

What do you do?_____

_____

_____

_____
_____
_____

Enter the payment for $50.

Mr. Knose also insists there is an error on his statement. He says he wrote a check for $75 on January 30, but only $50 was credited to his family's accounts. Your response:

_____
_____
_____
_____
_____

Item
129. ☐ **T**he HMO that CHS has signed up with has sent a new copy of their contract (Document 41). Read through the contract then put it with the other contracts.

Item
130. ☐ **L**ee Galbrief walks into the office and hands you a subpoena for the records (both medical and billing records) of one of Dr. Sickman's patients. What do you do?

_____
_____
_____
_____
_____

Item
131. ☐ **N**umerous claims suddenly appear in your IN box. The following claim information was received from Dr. Butch M. N. Hackim, Surgeon. Enter the charges into the system.

CLAIM 61

Laminectomy with myelotomy ($2,160) performed on 2/13/XX on Ian N. Theroad at CHS Community Hospital. An SSO was performed by Dr. Peter Prussia. Diagnosis: Herniated Disk as result of auto accident (2/9/XX). First Visit: 2/9/XX. Patient Hospitalized: 2/9/XX to 2/21/XX.

CLAIM 62

Ian N. Theroad was involved in an auto accident on 2/9/XX which resulted in crushing injuries and multiple fractures of the right leg. Efforts to save the leg have been unsuccessful due to the spread of gangrene. On 2/17/XX the right leg was amputated at the thigh ($1,200). High complexity follow-up visits were performed on 2/18/XX, 2/19/XX, and 2/21/XX ($150 each).

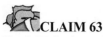

CLAIM 63

Hugh Waite has a history of morbid exogenous obesity. He is five feet eight inches tall and weighs 350 pounds. No matter what diet he tries, he can't seem to find a way to lose the weight. Finally he has decided to resort to drastic measures. A detailed admission ($250) was taken on 2/4/XX. Gastric stapling non vertical ($1,710) was performed on 2/5/XX. Extended hospital visits on 2/6/XX ($140) and 2/7/XX ($140), and a hospital discharge on 2/8/XX ($175). Date of first visit: 11/16/PY.

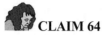

CLAIM 64

On 2/9/XX, Juana Fore-Theroad received a complex repair of a 5.1 cm. neck laceration ($330), a complex repair of a 2.1 cm. facial laceration ($240), removal of a portion of the steering wheel which was embedded in her jaw bone ($200), interdental fixation treatment of a jaw fracture ($1,000), treatment (with stabilization) of a fractured nasal bone ($170), and open treatment of a depressed fracture of the zygomatic arch ($485).

CLAIM 65

Juana Fore-Theroad received a modification of the lateral cartilage of nose ($1,195) at CHS Community Hospital on 2/16/XX. Ethmoidectomy, intra anterior ($620) and submucous resection turbinate, partial ($230) were performed on 2/12/XX. Diagnosis: Fracture nasal bones/fracture nasal septum, hemorrhagic sinusitis, hypertrophic turbinates. Date of accident: 2/9/XX.

Item 132. ☐ **M**rs. Baker calls up and says that she needs to schedule surgery for her 19-year-old daughter, Betsy. The surgery is elective and can be put off for a few months if it is convenient for the doctor. Mrs. Baker says she would like to schedule the surgery for two months from now. That way she can deal with her daughter's graduation from high school and birthday first, then handle the surgery after that. What do you say?

_____

_____

_____

_____

_____

_____

Item 133. ☐ **T**he following claim information was received from Dr. Will Kutteroff, Surgeon. Enter the charges into the system.

CLAIM 66

D.I. Dunnitt received a radial keratotomy ($1,100) on 2/4/XX in the outpatient department of CHS Community Hospital. Diagnosis: Degenerative Myopia.

CLAIM 67

On 2/10/XX, Kent C. Theroad was seen by Dr. Kutteroff for closed treatment of an ulna fracture ($390). A hospital discharge visit was also performed ($115).

CLAIM 68

Jose Fraide received a corpus callostomy ($2,950) on 02/06/XX. Detailed follow-up visits were performed on 02/07/XX and 02/08/XX ($85 ea). A discharge visit was performed on 02/09/XX ($115). Diagnosis: Epilepsy.

CLAIM 69

Carla Poole received a comprehensive consultation of moderate complexity ($275) on 2/1/XX. It was determined that she needed a bone cyst excised from the humerus ($910) and an excision of olecranon bursa ($255). These were done at CHS Community Hospital's outpatient department on 2/7/XX. Carla was referred by Dr. Sickman. Diagnosis: Tennis Elbow, Bursitis of Elbow.

CLAIM 70

Ian N. Theroad was involved in an auto accident on 2/9/XX. Once Ian was stabilized he was taken to the operating room for open treatment of a femoral shaft fracture with plate, screws, and cerclage ($1,560), and closed treatment of a skull fracture without operation ($95).

Item
134. ☐ **T**he following claim information was received from Dr. Ben Looney, Psychiatrist. Enter the charges into the system.

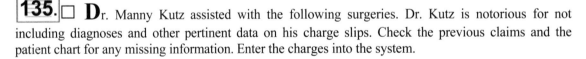

CLAIM 71

Codie Pendent received individual psychotherapy performed in the office on 2/4/XX, 2/13/XX, 2/20/XX, and 2/27/XX ($160 each). Diagnosis: Adjustment Disorder.

☞ Remember to fill out the authorized visits chart for any psychiatric treatments received by Codie Pendent.

Item
135. ☐ **D**r. Manny Kutz assisted with the following surgeries. Dr. Kutz is notorious for not including diagnoses and other pertinent data on his charge slips. Check the previous claims and the patient chart for any missing information. Enter the charges into the system.

CLAIM 72

Open treatment of a femoral shaft fracture with plate, screws, and cerclage ($460) on Ian N. Theroad on 2/9/XX.

CLAIM 73

A laminectomy with myelotomy ($430) on 2/13/XX on Ian N. Theroad.

CLAIM 74

An amputation of the right leg at the thigh on Ian N. Theroad, 2/17/XX ($275).

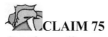

CLAIM 75

Gastric stapling non-vertical ($350) on 2/5/XX on Hugh Waite.

CLAIM 76

Complex repair of a 5.1 cm. neck laceration ($85), a complex repair of a 2.1 cm. facial laceration ($50), interdental fixation treatment of a jaw fracture ($200), and removal of a one cm. foreign body from the jaw bone ($55), treatment (with stabilization) of a fractured nasal bone ($50), and open treatment of a depressed fracture of the zygomatic arch ($100) performed on Juana Fore-Theroad on 2/9/XX.

CLAIM 77

Ethmoidectomy, intra anterior ($125) and submucous resection turbinate, partial ($50) were performed on 2/12/XX. Reconstruction of the lateral cartilage of nose ($240) performed on Juana Fore-Theroad on 2/16/XX.

CLAIM 78

Capsulotomy, extensive, including posterior ($400) performed on P'Lisa Waite on 1/8/XX.

CLAIM 79

Cholecystectomy with exploration of common duct ($350) performed on Petey Attricks at CHS Community Hospital on 1/15/XX.

CLAIM 80

Corpus callostomy ($600) on 02/06/XX on Jose Fraide.

CLAIM 81

Complete stripping of long, saphenous vein ($125) performed on Sherry Attricks on 2/1/XX.

CLAIM 82

Hysterectomy ($150), oophorectomy ($250), a laparoscopy with lysis of adhesions ($65), and dilation of vagina under anesthesia ($35) were performed on Cass N. O'Gen on 2/12/XX. Diagnosis: Left Ovarian Mass, Pelvic Adhesions, Severe Recto-Cystocele.

Item 136. ☐ You discover that Paul A. Mussel, a patient, has two insurance coverages and you listed the primary payor as secondary and vice versa. The secondary payor has just paid the claim as if they were primary. What do you do?

_____

_____

_____

_____

_____

_____

Item 137. ☐ **D**r. Anne S. Thesia, Anesthesiologist, provided anesthesia during the following operations. Enter these charges into the system.

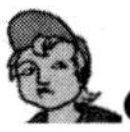

CLAIM 83

Amputation of right leg at thigh on Ian N. Theroad on 2/17/XX, emergency conditions ($2,500). Diagnosis: Multiple Fractures, Gangrene. Total anesthesia time: 0945 - 1420.

CLAIM 84

Epidural anesthesia for Jeanette Akenja-Nearing during labor and vaginal delivery on 2/25/XX ($1,950) (Dr. Thesia was not continuously present). Total anesthesia time: 8 hours 25 minutes.

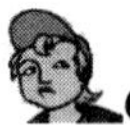

CLAIM 85

A laminectomy with myelotomy ($3,000) performed on 2/13/XX on Ian N. Theroad. Diagnosis: Herniated Disk as result of auto accident on 2/9/XX. Total anesthesia time: 2 hours 25 minutes.

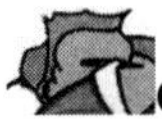

CLAIM 86

Gastric stapling non-vertical ($2,800) performed on Hugh Waite on 2/5/XX. Diagnosis: Morbid Exogenous Obesity. Total anesthesia time: 4 hours 20 minutes.

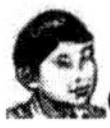

CLAIM 87

Radial Keratotomy ($1,800) performed on D.I. Dunnitt on 2/4/XX. Diagnosis: Degenerative Myopia. Total anesthesia time: 1710 - 1805.

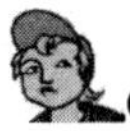

CLAIM 88

Open treatment of a femoral shaft fracture with plate, screws, and cerclage ($2,500), and closed treatment of a skull fracture without operation ($150) performed on Ian N. Theroad on 2/9/XX. Total anesthesia time: 2120 - 0115. Emergency conditions.

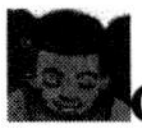

CLAIM 89

Excision of bone cyst from the humerus ($1,890) and an excision of olecranon bursa ($250) performed on Carla Poole on 2/7/XX. Diagnosis: Tennis Elbow, Bursitis of Elbow. Total anesthesia time: Start 8:50. Stop 12:35.

Item 138. ☐ **M**rs. I. Sawit, an elderly patient, calls up and asks for an immediate appointment, stating that she thinks she has kidney failure. She indicates that last night there was a television program about a woman with kidney failure and the symptoms the woman was listing sounds exactly like those she is experiencing. This is the third time she has requested an appointment after seeing a television program about a certain disease. What do you do?

_____

_____

_____

_____

_____

_____

Item
139. ☐ **R**eturn to entering the claims from Dr. Anne S. Thesia.

CLAIM 90

Reconstruction of the lateral cartilage of nose ($3,125) performed on Juana Fore-Theroad on 2/16/XX. Ethmoidectomy, intra anterior ($500) and submucous resection turbinate, partial ($350) performed on 2/12/XX. Diagnosis: Fracture nasal bones/fracture nasal septum, hemorrhagic sinusitis, hypertrophic turbinates. Total anesthesia time: 16:45 - 18:30 on 2/12/XX and 13:20 - 16:10 on 2/16/XX.

CLAIM 91

Complex repair of a 5.1 cm. neck laceration ($500), a complex repair of a 2.1 cm. facial laceration ($350), removal of 1 cm. foreign body in jaw with interdental fixation treatment of a jaw fracture ($1,200), treatment (with stabilization) of a fractured nasal bone ($250), and open treatment of a depressed fracture of the zygomatic arch ($450) performed on Juana Fore-Theroad on 2/9/XX. Monitoring of blood gases ($95). Total anesthesia time: 10:15 - 14:05. Emergency conditions.

CLAIM 92

Vaginal hysterectomy with oophorectomy ($2,850) performed on Cass N. O'Gen on 2/12/XX. Diagnosis: Left ovarian mass, pelvic adhesions, severe recto-cystocele. Total anesthesia time: 16:10 - 19:25.

CLAIM 93

Anesthesia for a corpus callostomy ($2,800) on Jose Fraide on 02/06/XX. Time: 12:00 – 3:15

Item
140. ☐ **R**hea E. Bright, Radiologist, performed the following on 2/9/XX. Enter these charges into the system.

CLAIM 94

On Juana Fore-Theroad: x-rays of facial bones (3 views) ($50), skull (5 views w/o stereo) ($85), and cervical spine ($40). Diagnosis: Zygomatic arch fx, jaw fx, nasal fx, concussion.

CLAIM 95

On Kent C. Theroad: x-ray of left arm (ulna, 3 views) ($30). Diagnosis: Ulna Fx.

CLAIM 96

On Ian N. Theroad: MRI of the right leg ($700) and x-rays of the skull (six views w/stereo) ($85), full spine ($65), right and left leg (a/p & lat of femur and tibia/fibula) ($40 each), and both arms (a/p & lat of both upper and lower rat and let arm) ($35 each). Diagnosis: crushed right leg, skull fix, multiple contusions, auto accident.

Item

141. ☐ **M**r. Al K. Holic, a patient, comes in with his bill and says that you did not bill it correctly. He was treated for a laceration above the right eye. He states that some drunk guy hit him in a bar, and the other guy started the fight. It was not his fault and therefore it should be considered an accident. What do you do?

_____

_____

_____

_____

_____

_____

Item
142. ☐ **T**he following claim information was received from Dr. Phil Goode. Enter these charges into the system.

 CLAIM 97

Dr. Goode performed a comprehensive exam of high complexity ($190) on Pat O'Gen in the office on 2/9/XX. Dr. Goode found the patient to have a cystic lesion of the left-upper eyelid and performed an outpatient excision of lesion with flap reconstruction, eyelid ($1,135) at CHS Community Hospital outpatient department on 2/12/XX. A follow-up exam problem focused ($65) was done on 2/16/XX. A dressing tray ($50) was used on 2/12/XX.

Item
143. ☐ **Y**ou take a break and go out to a nearby deli. On your way back, while standing in the lobby waiting for the elevator, you overhear Mr. Arthur Ritus, a middle aged patient, talking on the phone. He says that he is being treated by another doctor, as well as Dr. Goode. When you check his records, there is no indication of this. What do you do?

_____

_____

_____

_____

_____

Item
144. ☐ **T**he following claim information was received from Dr. Yu B. Sickman. Enter these charges into the system.

 CLAIM 98

Ova Waite has been playing too much golf lately and one of her ribs has become very sore. She expected the tenderness to go down, but it hasn't. Mrs. Waite received an office visit with straightforward decision making ($55) in the office on 1/18/XX. An injection of tendon sheath ($90) was also performed on 1/18/XX. On 2/17/XX the patient came back to the office and Dr. Sickman performed arthrocentesis on the elbow ($90). Diagnosis: Neuralgia/neuritis, Costochondritis.

CLAIM 99

Sherry Attricks requested surgery for varicose veins of the right leg. A complete stripping of long, saphenous vein ($600) was performed on 2/1/XX by Dr. Yu B. Sickman at the outpatient department of CHS Community Hospital. On 2/12/XX an injection of solution (multiple) into telangiectasia ($240) was performed by Dr. Sickman at the office. (No SSO performed.)

CLAIM 100

Scarlet Fever has not been feeling well since she went hiking with her family on 1/21/XX. She is weak with muscular aches and severe headaches and chills. On 1/28/XX, Dr. Sickman performed an office visit of high complexity ($190), CBC ($20), and WBC (manual) ($20). Dr. Sickman also gave her an injection of antibiotics ($30). Diagnosis: Rocky Mountain Spotted Fever. Patient was admitted to CHS Community Hospital.

CLAIM 101

Dr. Sickman performed a high complexity hospital visit on Scarlet Fever on 1/29/XX, 1/30/XX, 1/31/XX, and 2/1/XX ($130 each). He also administered IV infusion of antibiotic for less than one hour on 1/29/XX ($143). A hospital discharge was performed on 2/2/XX ($115). Diagnosis: Rocky Mountain Spotted Fever.

CLAIM 102

Mrs. Fraide came into the office on 01/15/XX with her son Jose, who has epilepsy. It appears that the current medications are not working. Jose received a high complexity exam ($190), a CBC ($30) and a urinalysis ($30). Symptoms began 02/28/PY. A copayment of $15 was made for this visit (see Window Payments section).

CLAIM 103

Jose Fraide was seen in the office on 02/03/XX for additional testing to determine if he was a likely candidate for surgical treatment. Tests included a head CT ($350), skull x-ray ($80) and MRI of the skull ($800). A full metabolic panel ($30) was also performed. Diagnosis: Epilepsy. A copayment of $15 was made for this visit. (see Window Payments section).

CLAIM 104

Mrs. Fraide brought Jose into Dr. Sickman's office on 02/25/XX. Jose received a detailed office visit of moderate complexity ($115). It appears the surgery has helped to drastically reduce the number of seizures Jose experiences. Diagnosis: Epilepsy. A copayment of $15 was made for this visit. (see Window Payments section).

Item 145. ☐ **Y**ou receive a phone call from Andy Pendent: "Hi, I'm Andy Pendent. I'm Codie Pendent's husband and Dee's father. We've moved recently and I wanted to make sure we would be getting our bills. Can you tell me what address you have on your records?" What do you do or say?

_____

_____

_____

_____

_____

Item 146. ☐ **S**omething is going on with Dee Pendent. What is it and what should you do about it?

_____

_____

_____

_____

_____

_____

Item 147. ☐ **Y**ou receive an EOMB for charges with Medicare (Document 42). Enter the payments on the appropriate patient records, calculate the write-off amount and enter it (☞) onto the patient's ledger card or (🖥) into the computer. Then balance bill the appropriate party, either additional insurance or the patient if necessary.

Item 148. ☐ **Y**ou receive a notice from Medicare. One of the services for Shay Kee Hart has been determined "Not medically necessary." You had collected money for the patient's portion of services. What do you do about this?

_____

_____

_____

_____

_____

_____

Item 149. ☐ **T**he following claim information was received from CHS Medical Supply. Their information is:

CHS Medical Supply
9882 Clinton Ave.
Colter, CO 81222
Phone: (970) 555-9100
EIN: 40-8761234
Enter these charges into the system.

CLAIM 105

Upon the order of Dr. Sickman, a glucometer was purchased for $273 by Candy Dunnitt on 1/21/XX. Diagnosis: Diabetes Mellitus.

CLAIM 106

Because of D. Jobb Dunnitt's diagnosis of chronic bronchitis per Dr. Goode, a nebulizer with compressor was rented at $127.50 per month from 1/1/XX to 3/1/XX.

CLAIM 107

On the order of Dr. Pulse, an apnea monitor ($175) was purchased for Wade N. Poole on 3/1/XX. Diagnosis: Apnea. Date of first symptom: 3/1/XX.

CLAIM 108

On the order of Dr. Sickman, an orthotic (foot stabilizer) left foot - Phelps ($397) was purchased for P'Lisa Waite on 1/9/XX. Diagnosis: Clubfoot.

CLAIM 109

On the order of Dr. Goode, a juvenile wheelchair ($1,324) was purchased for Beane Andy Knose on 1/3/XX. Diagnosis: Cerebral Palsy.

Item 150. ☐ **W**hen entering a patient's claim you routinely check their chart. You are sure Sig Natur, a new patient, signed a "Right to Release Information" slip, but it is not in his file and you cannot find it. The office manager is pressuring you to send in the claim for payment as soon as possible. What do you do?

_____

_____

_____

_____

_____

_____

Item 151. ☐ **T**he following claims were received from CHS Ambulance service. Their information is:

CHS Ambulance Service
1389 Castle Blvd.
Colter, CO 81222
Phone: (970) 555-9111
EIN: 40-1478523

Enter these charges into the system.

CLAIM 110

Upon arrival at the home of Candy Dunnitt on 2/16/XX, patient was in a diabetic coma. Patient was transported from 160 Abernathy Avenue, Apt. #A, Armstrong, CO 81569 and taken to CHS Community Hospital in an ambulance with advance life support ($527). Diagnosis: Diabetes Mellitus.

CLAIM 111

D. Jobb Dunnitt was transported with EKG monitoring from 160 Abernathy Ave., Apt. #A, Armstrong, CO 81569 to CHS Community Hospital on 1/9/XX ($348). Pt was suffering from chest pains.

CLAIM 112

On 2/9/XX, Kent C. Theroad and Donette Theroad were jointly transported from Interstate 70 (zip code 81232) to CHS Community Hospital, 12 miles ($272 each). Diagnosis: Auto Accident.

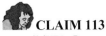 **CLAIM 113**

On 2/9/XX, Juana Fore-Theroad was transported with ALS from Interstate 70 (zip code 81232) to CHS Community Hospital, 12 miles ($423). Diagnosis: face and neck lacerations, puncture wound with embedded foreign body, lower right jaw, shock, auto accident.

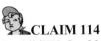 **CLAIM 114**

On 2/9/XX, Ian N. Theroad was transported by air ambulance from Interstate 70 (zip code 81232) to CHS Community Hospital, eight miles ($1,139). Crushed right thigh, multiple open fractures of right thigh, head injuries, shock, auto accident.

Item 152. ☐ **E**lle Darly is a patient who is covered by her employers plan. Her grandson, whom she takes care of, is her dependent on the plan. In 30 days Mrs. Darly will be turning 65 years old. Will this cause any changes to her insurance coverage? If so, what is it and what should you do about it?

_____

_____

_____

_____

_____

_____

Will it also affect her grandson? If so, in what way?_____

_____

_____

_____

_____

_____

Item 153. ☐ **P**rint or write up a day sheet or daily journal.

Item 154. ☐ **P**rint or write up a deposit slip for all monies received. Attach all checks and cash payments to it.

Item 155. ☐ **R**econcile petty cash. Count all money remaining in petty cash and be sure you have the same amount left at the end of the day as you started with at the beginning. If not, determine exactly where the missing amount is.

Item 156. ☐ Print all the claims you have entered today. If you are using one-part forms, print two copies (see following exercise).

Item 157. ☐ **P**repare claims for mailing. Place one copy of the claim in the patient file. Place the second copy together with all claims for a single carrier. Print or write address labels and attach them to the claims. Be sure to separate out any claims which are for secondary insurance. They should not be billed until the EOB is received from the first carrier.

Item 158. ☐ Print a transaction list report. Use 3/4/XX as the date of the report. The report should include all entries, so 01/01/XX-03/04/XX should be the range of dates. This will allow the computer to pick up all entries. Check your answers before proceeding. If there are any errors, correct them before proceeding.

Item 159. ☐ **M**rs. Gandmah calls up and says that her 17-year-old daughter recently came in for a pregnancy test and they were supposed to call back to get the results of that test today. You pull the patient's chart and find that the test was positive. You also notice that the patient is listed as married, and is still listed as a dependent on her father's medical insurance. What do you do?

_____

_____

_____

_____

_____

_____

Item 160. ☐ **D**. Jobb Dunnitt calls in. He says they just found out his son D.I. is allergic to Codeine and Valium. He would like this information added to the patient chart. Place a notation on the family's patient information sheet and (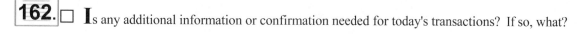) enter this information into the Patient Information screen.

Item 161. ☐ **P**atient statements for the month of February need to be mailed out.

☞ Make sure that all patient statements have been updated and are showing correct balances due. Make a copy of those that have balances of more than $1.

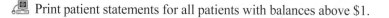 Print patient statements for all patients with balances above $1.

Item 162. ☐ **I**s any additional information or confirmation needed for today's transactions? If so, what?

_____

_____

_____

_____

Item 163. ☐ **S**top and check that all assignments are correct before continuing on to the next date.

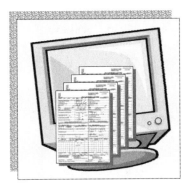

March 22, 20XX

Item 164. ☐ **T**oday's date is March 22, 20XX

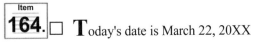 Change the date to: March 22, 20XX.

Item 165. ☐ **C**ount petty cash. How much is in the cash envelope? ....

Item 166. ☐ **O**n your desk you find a detailing of charges paid by Rover Insurers, Inc. (Document 43). Credit the appropriate amounts to the correct accounts, then do any balance billing to either the patient or an additional insurance carrier. When billing a secondary insurance payor, be sure to attach a copy of the EOB. Data for other patients should be redacted. A copy of the EOB need not be attached when you are balance billing the patient. The insurance carrier should have already sent them a copy of the EOB.

Item 167. ☐ **T**here is a note in Kent C. Theroad's file asking you to call him when the insurance payment comes in. You contact him and he states that his family was involved in an auto accident on 2/9/XX and he is sure that the family's portion of the expenses will be quite high. He asks to set up a payment plan for the amount they owe. What is the amount owed on each member of the family, after the insurance company has made payment (do not include charges which the insurance company has not yet made payment on)?

....

....

....

....

What is the total of the remaining amounts owed on the family's accounts? ....

Mr. Theroad suggests paying a $50 initial payment with additional payments of $25 per month. What is your response? ....

....

_____
_____
_____
_____
_____

Item 168. ☐ **U**sing the Payment Plan Letter in the back of the book, set up a payment plan with Mr. Theroad for an initial payment of $50 and $25 per month. Make a note on the payment agreement that this payment plan is valid only for the total shown on the page. Any additional payments due for other or continuing treatments will need to be covered under a separate payment plan, or services will need to be paid for at the time they are rendered.

Item 169. ☐ **S**ue Pervisor tells you to make a list of all accounts with balances past due. She tells you to make calls, write letters, or do whatever you have to do to collect on these accounts.

> ☞ Using the Patient Aging Form in the back of the book, make up a list of all patients with charges 30, 60, and 90 days past due. Write one sample collection letter for those with balances 30 and 60 days past due. Write a separate letter for those accounts which are 90 days or more past due.

> Print an aging report showing all balances past due 30 days or more. (Note: Some computer programs work off the internal date (windows date) on the computer. If this date has not been changed, charges may not show up in the appropriate past due columns. If this is the case with your computer program, use the Patient Aging Form in the back of the book.). Then write one sample collection letter for those with balances 30 and 60 days past due. Write a separate letter for those accounts which are 90 days or more past due.

Item 170. ☐ **D**r. Goode sends you a missed appointment charge ($25) for Mr. Don Comin, a patient with a case of uncontrolled hypertension. This is the third time he has missed his appointment. What do you do?

_____
_____
_____
_____
_____
_____

Item 171. ☐ **S**ue Pervisor asks you to give her $20 from petty cash for some small office supplies she needs to buy. She says to charge it to the supplies account, 6040. What do you do?

_____
_____
_____
_____
_____

Item 172. ☐ **Y**ou receive a phone call from Dr. Payne asking about the dates services were performed for any members of the O'Gen family and any payments related to these charges. Fill in the information below.

Date	Patient	Services Performed	Charges	Payment(s)

Total all charges and payments _____

Item 173. ☐ **D**r. Payne also asks you to estimate how much will be paid on each of these charges by the insurance carrier if the carrier has not yet made payment on the bill. Fill in your estimate of or the actual payment from the insurance carrier below. If you are estimating, show how you arrived at the estimate.

You call the insurance carrier and they tell you that their computers are down and will not be up until tomorrow. Use the insurance coverage sheet and the previous claims for this family to estimate how much deductible has been paid for each member of the family. Then estimate the patient's portion of the above charges.

	Deductible	Deductible Paid	Estimated Insurance Pmt.	Patient Amount
Pat				
Cass				
Ox				

If the insurance pays the amount estimated, how much will be remaining on the family's bills? _____

_____

Item 174. ☐ **D**r. Goode's receptionist calls and says she needs to contact the insurance carrier for Scarlet Fever. Write down the name, address, phone number, and policy name and/or number for the insurance carrier.

_____

_____

_____

_____

_____

_____

Item 175. ☐ **D**r. Hackim hands you a note regarding services he performed a couple days ago (Document 44). Evan Lee Harps was not a patient of this practice. Use the information you have to create a Patient Information Sheet and chart for Evan Lee Harps. Also bill the appropriate insurance carrier(s).

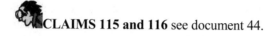 **CLAIMS 115 and 116** see document 44.

 The information you have regarding this patient will need to be entered into the computer system before billing for insurances can take place.

Item 176. ☐ **E**ach doctor needs to know which of his patients have amounts past due for services they rendered.

☞ Using the list you created in item 169, create a separate list for each doctor showing which patients have past due accounts.

 Print a patient aging report for all doctors.

Item 177. ☐ **D**r. Payne sends you a note stating she is writing off $50 from Cass N. O'Gen's bill due to financial hardship. She would also like to know how much is left to pay on this bill. Make an adjustment on the patient's records. (For audit purposes, be sure the adjustment contains information as to why this amount is being written off by using the new codes.) What is the amount remaining on Cass N. O'Gen's bill after adjustment?

_____

Item 178. ☐ **A**l Weighs Knose returns the statement for Beane Andy Knose's wheelchair purchase with a note written across the bottom: "Please bill my credit card for the balance due on the wheelchair." The following credit card information is given:

Credit Card Type & Number: _____ Visa 4444 3333 2222 1111 _____
Credit Card Name:___ Al Weighs Knose _____ Expiration Date:____ 3/10/XX _____

Add the credit card payment to his account, and add the credit card information to his patient record.

 Be sure to add the credit card information in the appropriate place on the patient information screen.

Item 179. ☐ **E**mma Barrased calls on the phone and asks to make an appointment with Dr. Payne as soon as possible. When you ask the purpose of the visit she becomes embarrassed and refuses to say. What do you do?

_____

_____

_____

_____

_____

_____

Item 180. ☐ **M**s. Penny Wise steps up to the window and indicates that she needs to make an advance payment on her daughter's surgery, which will take place on March 30th (10 days from now). She hands you a patient information sheet which states that she does not have insurance. The bill is expected to run $3,000 to $4,000. She wants to make an advance payment of $2,000. Both she and her husband work full-time and they should be able to make another payment within 30 days of the surgery. What do you do?

_____

_____

_____

_____

_____

Item 181. ☐ **A**l Weighs Knose calls in and says he has filed for bankruptcy. What do you do?

_____

_____

_____

_____

Item 182. ☐ **P**rint or write up a day sheet or daily journal.

Item 183. ☐ **P**rint or write up a deposit slip for all monies received. Attach all checks and cash payments to it.

Item 184. ☐ **R**econcile petty cash. Count all money remaining in petty cash and be sure you have the same amount left at the end of the day as you started with at the beginning. If not, determine exactly where the missing amount is.

Item 185. ☐ 🖥 Print all the claims you have entered today. If you are using one-part forms, print two copies (see following exercise).

Item 186. ☐ **P**repare claims for mailing. Place one copy of the claim in the patient file. Place the second copy together with all claims for a single carrier. Print or write address labels and attach them to the claims.

Item 187. ☐ 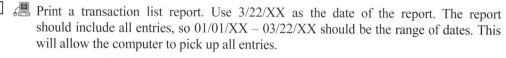 Print a transaction list report. Use 3/22/XX as the date of the report. The report should include all entries, so 01/01/XX – 03/22/XX should be the range of dates. This will allow the computer to pick up all entries.

Item 188. ☐ ☞ Make a list of all patients with balances above $5 who have not made a payment in the last week.

☐ Print statements for all patients with balances above $5 who have not made a payment in the last week.

Item 189. ☐ Print patient ledgers for all patients.

Item 190. ☐ Print a Practice Analysis report for the period from January 1 to the present for Drs. Goode and Sickman.

Item 191. ☐ **P**rint or write up an Insurance Analysis Report (Insurance Claims Register) for the period from January 1, 20XX to March 22, 20XX.

Item 192. ☐ **P**rint or write up an Insurance Aging Report for the period from January 1, 20XX to March 20, 20XX.

Item 193. ☐ **I**s any additional information or confirmation needed? If so, what?

_____

_____

_____

_____

_____

 Congratulations, you have now completed the simulated work portion of the course! You are now ready to prepare your resume and enter the exciting world of medical billing. **Good Luck!**

CLUES FOR SIMULATED WORK PROGRAM ASSIGNMENTS

The following clues may help you with the critical thinking exercises contained in the simulated work program. Before looking at these clues you should attempt to answer the question on your own. Then look at the clue and determine if you should revise your answer or if you are happy with it the way it is.

Item #   Clues

14.	What are the steps involved in obtaining treatment authorizations?
15.	Are any of these diagnoses work-related?
16.	Should you tell the doctor? What options are available for payments?
34.	Consider Medicare eligibility guidelines.
36.	What would Medicare say? Are there any legal ramifications to this arrangement?
37.	Can you still bill Medicare for these charges? What are the rules?
40.	What items might indicate the payment, if there was one?
43.	Are mumps communicable?
46.	Are there other clinical personnel (RN/LPN) available to triage this patient?
50.	Are there clinical personnel available to triage this patient?
52.	Are there any legal ramifications you should consider? What is the best way to handle this? What are the guidelines of his insurance carrier?
58.	Check the patient's insurance coverage.
60.	Is there a clinical person available to answer his questions? What about general available information? Other resources?
61.	Should you tell the doctor? What payment options are available? What other resources might there be?
62.	Remember privacy issues.
63.	In what cases would the insurance carrier pay the patient even if benefits are assigned?
70.	Would you need verification? How would you handle the patient's accounts?
77.	How could you find out what language it is? Where might you find other people who speak this language? Are there any written language resources available?
78.	Should you be concerned, even if her mother is not?
79.	What is the proper way to transfer a patient chart?
83.	How can you trace these people?
87.	What are the legal ramifications? How should you send the letter?
92.	Why might it make a difference what day the surgery is scheduled?
101.	How can you be sure that it arrives this time? Is there anyone you should talk to about the problem?
104.	Check the contract provisions. Is there any way to get coverage for a pre-existing condition? What makes a condition pre-existing?
105.	Remember privacy issues.
106.	Why might they think he is not covered when he is? What do you do if he is not covered?
121.	At what point does an honest mistake become fraud?
124.	Whom should you seek reimbursement from?
125.	How can you get the money and still make the patient feel good about the provider?
126.	In what case might only one deductible be taken on claims for several family members?
128.	What happens if you cash the check as it is? Check all documentation. Whose mistake is it?
130.	What are the legal ramifications of turning over the records? Of not turning over the records?
132.	Why might it make a difference what day the surgery is scheduled?
136.	How can you verify the accuracy of each carrier's payment?

138. Is there a clinical person available to triage her call?
141. What are the rules governing this situation? How or why might the patient know these rules?
143. What are the medical implications of this situation? Who needs to know about this, if anyone?
145. Remember privacy issues.
146. What is a condyloma? How do you get it? What are her other doctor visits for?
148. Is there anything in the Medicare agreement the provider signed governing this situation?
150. What are the legal implications of sending it in? Of not sending it in?
152. Check the patient's insurance coverage.
159. Can a married person be a dependent on a parent's insurance policy? What do the contracts in this book say? Should you give the mother the test results?
167. How will these payments affect the principal and/or interest on the account?
170. Are there any legal concerns regarding his missing appointments for this diagnosis?
171. Does Sue Pervisor have the authority to take money from petty cash? What does it say in the front of this book under petty cash?
179. Why might you (or the doctor) need to know the reason for the visit?
180. From where do most people obtain insurance coverage? Why might they say that they don't have insurance? If they have no insurance, how can you be sure of getting the remaining amount on the surgery in a timely manner?
181. Now what happens with his accounts? Can you still collect the money?

Documents

Documents

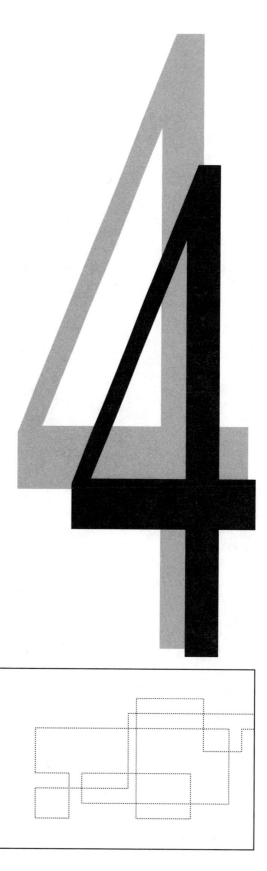

Document 1

PATIENT INFORMATION SHEET

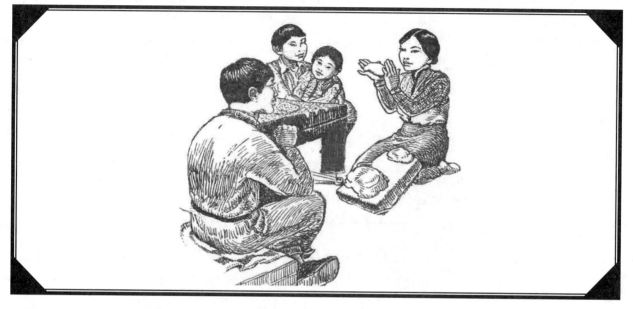

INSURED'S INFORMATION

Patient ID: _DDU5501-001_   Assigned Provider: _Dr. Phil Goode_   Birth date: _Apr. 4, 1967_

Name: (Last, First, Middle) _Dunnitt, D. Jobb_   Sex: _Male_

Address: (Inc City, State, Zip) _160 Abernathy Ave. Apt #A, Armstrong, CO 81569_

Home Phone: _(970) 555-1122_   Marital Status: _Widowed_   Social Security #: _111-11-1111_

Employer Name: _White Corporation - Demolitions Team_   Work Phone: _(970) 555-1234_

Employer Address: _1234 Whitaker Lane, Colter, CO 81250_

Employment Status: _Full-Time_   Referred by: _Friend - Amanda Alexander_

Allergies/Medical conditions: _Bronchitis_

Primary Ins Name: _Winter Insurance Co._   Address: _9763 Western Way, Whittier, CO 82963_

ID #: _111-11-Whi_   Plan #/Name: _White Corp._   Policy Holder Name: _D. Jobb Dunnitt_

Secondary Ins Name: _N/A_   Address: _____

ID #: _____   Plan #/Name: _____   Policy Holder Name: _____

SPOUSE'S INFORMATION

Patient ID: _____   Assigned Provider: _____   Birth date: _____

Name: (Last, First, Middle) _N/A_   Sex: _____

Social Security #: _____   Employment Status: _____

Employer Name: _____   Work Phone: _____

Employer Address: _____

Allergies/Medical conditions: _____

Primary Ins Name: _____   Address: _____

ID #: _____   Plan #/Name: _____   Policy Holder Name: _____

Secondary Ins Name: _____   Address: _____

ID #: _____   Plan #/Name: _____   Policy Holder Name: _____

CHILD #1

Patient ID: _CDU5502-002_   Assigned Provider: _Dr. Phil Goode_   Birth date: _Apr. 16, 1991_

Name of Minor Child: _Dunnitt, Candy_   Social Security #: _104-16-1984_

Sex: _Female_   Marital Status: _Single_   Relationship to Insured: _Daughter_

Allergies/Medical conditions: _Diabetes_

Primary Ins Name: _Winter Insurance Co._   Primary Insured: _Father_

Secondary Ins Name: _N/A_   Secondary Insured: _____

CHILD #2

Patient ID: _DDU5503-003_   Assigned Provider: _Dr. Phil Goode_   Birth date: _Aug. 24, 1993_

Name of Minor Child: _Dunnitt, D.I._   Social Security #: _108-24-1986_

Sex: _Male_   Marital Status: _Single_   Relationship to Insured: _Son_

Allergies/Medical conditions: _____

Primary Ins Name: _Winter Insurance Co._   Primary Insured: _Father_

Secondary Ins Name: _N/A_   Secondary Insured: _____

CHILD #3

Patient ID: _VDU5504-004_   Assigned Provider: _Dr. Phil Goode_   Birth date: _Oct. 16, 1995_

Name of Minor Child: _Dunnitt, V. Iris_   Social Security #: _110-16-1988_

Sex: _Female_   Marital Status: _Single_   Relationship to Insured: _Daughter_

Allergies/Medical conditions: _____

Primary Ins Name: _Winter Insurance Co._   Primary Insured: _Father_

Secondary Ins Name: _N/A_   Secondary Insured: _____

EMERGENCY CONTACT

Name: _D. Boss_   Home Phone: _(970) 555-8890_   Other Phone: _(970) 555-6031_

Address: (Inc City, State, Zip) _4310 Nowayout St., Armstrong, CO 81569_

ACKNOWLEDGMENT AND AUTHORITY FOR TREATMENT AND PAYMENT

_DD_   I consent to treatment as necessary or desirable to the care of the patient named above, including but not restricted to whatever drugs, medicine, performance of operations and conduct of laboratory, x-ray, or other studies that may be used by the attending doctor, his/her nurse or qualified designate:

_DD_   I also acknowledge full responsibility for the payment of such services and agree to pay for them upon demand, in full, AT THE TIME OF SERVICE. If the physician must use a collection agency/attorney or court to collect its charges, then I will pay reasonable attorney fees and costs incurred in collecting same, regardless of insurance coverage.

_DD_   I hereby authorize payment directly to Consolidated Health Services of the medical expense benefits otherwise payable to me but not to exceed my indebtedness to said physician on account of the enclosed charge.

_DD_   I hereby authorize any medical practitioner, medical or medically related facility, insurance or reinsuring company, consumer reporting agency, or employer having information with respect to any physical or mental condition and/or treatment of me or my minor children and any other non-medical information of me and my minor children to give to the group policy holder, my employer, or its legal representative, any and all such information.

_DD_   I understand the information obtained by the use of the Authorization will be used to determine eligibility for insurance, and eligibility for benefits under any existing policy. Any information obtained will not be released by/to any organization EXCEPT to the group policyholder, my employer, reinsuring companies, the Medical Information Bureau, Inc., or other persons or organizations performing business or legal services in connection with my application, claim, or as may be otherwise lawfully required or as I may further authorize.

_DD_   I further agree that a photographic copy of this Authorization shall be valid as the original. This Authorization shall be valid for one year from the date shown below.

Signature of Insured: _D. Job Dunnitt_   Date: _Jan. 9, 20XX_

Signature of Spouse: _____   Date: _____

PATIENT INFORMATION SHEET

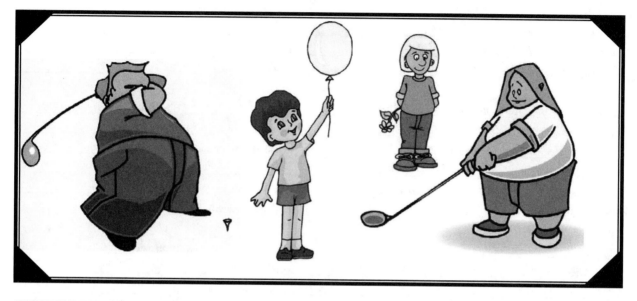

INSURED'S INFORMATION

Patient ID: __HWA5505-005__ Assigned Provider: _____ Birth date: _Jul. 10, 1970_

Name: (Last, First, Middle) __Waite, Hugh__ Sex: __Male__

Address: (Inc City, State, Zip) _222 Barker Blvd., Colter, CO 81222_

Home Phone: _(970) 555-2211_ Marital Status: _Married_ Social Security #: _222-11-2222_

Employer Name: __Blue Corporation__ Work Phone: _(970) 555-9876 x561_

Employer Address: _9817 Bobcat Blvd., Bastion, CO 81319_

Employment Status: __Full-time__ Referred by: _____

Allergies/Medical conditions: _____

Primary Ins Name: _Ball Insurance Carriers_ Address: _3895 Bubble Blvd., Ste. 283, Boxwood, CO 85931_

ID #: _222-11-2222_ Plan #/Name: _98135 Blue_ Policy Holder Name: _Huge Waite_

Secondary Ins Name: __N/A__ Address: _____

ID #: _____ Plan #/Name: _____ Policy Holder Name: _____

SPOUSE'S INFORMATION

Patient ID: __OWA5506-006__ Assigned Provider: _____ Birth date: _May 15, 1973_

Name: (Last, First, Middle) __Waite, Ova__ Sex: __Female__

Social Security #: _221-93-2495_ Employment Status: _Homemaker_

Employer Name: _____ Work Phone: _____

Employer Address: _____

Allergies/Medical conditions: _____

Primary Ins Name: _See Husband_ Address: _____

ID #: _____ Plan #/Name: _____ Policy Holder Name: _____

Secondary Ins Name: _____ Address: _____

ID #: _____ Plan #/Name: _____ Policy Holder Name: _____

CHILD #1

Patient ID: ___PWA5507-007___ Assigned Provider: _____ Birth date: *Mar. 11, 1999*

Name of Minor Child: ___*Waite, P'Lisa*___ Social Security #: _198-80-3112_

Sex: *Female* Marital Status: ___*Single*___ Relationship to Insured: *Daughter*

Allergies/Medical conditions: ___*Clubfoot*___

Primary Ins Name: *Ball Insurance Carriers* Primary Insured: __*Father*__

Secondary Ins Name: ___*N/A*___ Secondary Insured: _____

CHILD #2

Patient ID: ___DWA5508-008___ Assigned Provider: _____ Birth date: *June 5, 2000*

Name of Minor Child: __*Ben Waite*__ Social Security #: _555-85-5201_

Sex: ___*Male*___ Marital Status: ___*Single*___ Relationship to Insured: ___*Son*___

Allergies/Medical conditions: _____

Primary Ins Name: ___*Ball Insurance Carriers*___ Primary Insured: ___*Father*___

Secondary Ins Name: __*N/A*__ Secondary Insured: _____

CHILD #3

Patient ID: _____ Assigned Provider: _____ Birth date: _____

Name of Minor Child: _____ Social Security #: _____

Sex: _____ Marital Status: _____ Relationship to Insured: _____

Allergies/Medical conditions: _____

Primary Ins Name: _____ Primary Insured: _____

Secondary Ins Name: _____ Secondary Insured: _____

EMERGENCY CONTACT

Name: __*Imma Bigtoo*__ Home Phone: *(970) 555- 9080* Other Phone: *(970) 555- 6837*

Address: (Inc City, State, Zip)___*563 Blubber Road, Colter, CO 81222*___

ACKNOWLEDGMENT AND AUTHORITY FOR TREATMENT AND PAYMENT

___HW___ I consent to treatment as necessary or desirable to the care of the patient named above, including but not restricted to whatever drugs, medicine, performance of operations and conduct of laboratory, x-ray, or other studies that may be used by the attending doctor, his/her nurse or qualified designate:

___HW___ I also acknowledge full responsibility for the payment of such services and agree to pay for them upon demand, in full, AT THE TIME OF SERVICE. If the physician must use a collection agency/attorney or court to collect its charges, then I will pay reasonable attorney fees and costs incurred in collecting same, regardless of insurance coverage.

___HW___ I hereby authorize payment directly to Consolidated Health Services of the medical expense benefits otherwise payable to me but not to exceed my indebtedness to said physician on account of the enclosed charge.

___HW___ I hereby authorize any medical practitioner, medical or medically related facility, insurance or reinsuring company, consumer reporting agency, or employer having information with respect to any physical or mental condition and/or treatment of me or my minor children and any other non-medical information of me and my minor children to give to the group policy holder, my employer, or its legal representative, any and all such information.

___HW___ I understand the information obtained by the use of the Authorization will be used to determine eligibility for insurance, and eligibility for benefits under any existing policy. Any information obtained will not be released by/to any organization EXCEPT to the group policyholder, my employer, reinsuring companies, the Medical Information Bureau, Inc., or other persons or organizations performing business or legal services in connection with my application, claim, or as may be otherwise lawfully required or as I may further authorize.

___HW___ I further agree that a photographic copy of this Authorization shall be valid as the original. This Authorization shall be valid for one year from the date shown below.

Signature of Insured: __*Hugh Waite*__ Date: _*Jan. 11, 20XX*_

Signature of Spouse: __*Ova Waite*__ Date: _*Jan. 11, 20XX*_

Document 3

PROVIDER INFORMATION

1. Provider: Allota Payne, M.D., OB-GYN
    Address: 1357 Castle Blvd, Ste. 500, Colter, CO 81222
    Phone: (970) 555-5123
    License #:   AA163615
    EIN: 40-2233445
    MCR UPIN: AMP006
    Provider Accepts Medicare Assignment

2. Provider: Phil Goode, M.D.
    Address: 1357 Castle Blvd, Ste. 501B, Colter, CO 81222
    Phone: (970) 555-8425
    License #:   BB646545
    EIN: 40-2224096
    MCR UPIN: PRG007
    Provider Does Not Accept Medicare Assignment

3. Provider: Rhea E. Bright, M.D., Radiologist
    Address: 1357 Castle Blvd, Ste. 502, Colter, CO 81222
    Phone: (970) 555-7782
    License #:   CC4242342
    EIN: 40-3896529
    MCR UPIN: REB006
    Provider Accepts Medicare Assignment

4. Provider: CHS Community Hospital
    Address: 9876 Clinton Ave, Colter, CO 81222
    Phone: (970) 555-9215
    License #:   HO456565
    EIN: 40-9999999
    MCR UPIN: CCH620
    Provider Accepts Medicare Assignment

Provider #4 should also be entered into the address information screen, since doctors may provide services at this facility. Go into the Address Information screen. Use the address code CHS.

5. Provider: Ben Looney, M.D., Psychiatrist
    Address: 1357 Castle Blvd, Ste. 503, Colter, CO 81222
    Phone: (970) 555-2145
    License #:   DD484834
    EIN: 40-6666666
    MCR UPIN: BVL001
    Provider Accepts Medicare Assignment

6. Provider: Noah Pulse, M.D., ER
    Address: 2468 Castle Blvd, Ste. 612, Colter, CO 81222
    Phone: (970) 555-4656
    License #:   EE155313
    EIN: 40-9475245
    MCR UPIN: NDP076
    Provider Accepts Medicare Assignment

OFFICE VISIT PROCEDURES

DESCRIPTION	TIME	CHARGE	CPT® CODE	COST
NEW PATIENT OFFICE VISITS				
Problem focused history/exam, straightforward	20 min	$ 65	_____	0
Expanded history/exam, straightforward	30 min	$ 85	_____	0
Detailed history/exam, low complexity	40 min	$105	_____	0
Comprehensive history/exam, moderate complexity	45 min	$115	_____	0
Comprehensive history/exam, high complexity	60 min	$135	_____	0
ESTABLISHED PATIENT OFFICE VISITS				
Minimal visit	10 min	$ 35	_____	0
Problem focused history/exam, straightforward	15 min	$ 55	_____	0
Expanded history/exam, low complexity	20 min	$ 65	_____	0
Detailed history/exam, moderate complexity	25 min	$ 80	_____	0
Comprehensive history/exam, high complexity	30 min	$ 95	_____	0
Matrixectomy	30 min	$200	_____	45
EKG, 12 leads c/interp & report	20 min	$100	_____	15
Direction/Overseeing of emergency medical systems	15 min	$ 65	_____	10
Urinalysis	5 min	$ 30	_____	5
Specimen handling fee	5 min	$ 15	_____	0
Removal of .5 cm skin mole on neck with biopsy	45 min	$400	_____	30

ICD-9 CODES

Code the following diagnoses and enter the information into the Diagnosis Information screen. If necessary, add in additional descriptive information regarding the diagnosis.

	CODE	OFFICIAL CPT® DESCRIPTION
Abrasions, leg	_____	_____
Acute UTI	_____	_____
Broken Medial Ulna	_____	_____
Chest Pain	_____	_____
Chicken Pox	_____	_____
Clubfoot, congenital	_____	_____
Chronic Bronchitis	_____	_____
Concussion	_____	_____
Contusions, head	_____	_____
Cut Finger	_____	_____
Diabetes Mellitus	_____	_____
Flu	_____	_____
Gangrene	_____	_____
Hemorrhoids	_____	_____
Hyperlipidemia	_____	_____
Mole (skin), neck	_____	_____
Ovarian Mass	_____	_____
Pelvic Pain	_____	_____
Pelvis Adhesions	_____	_____
Pilonidal Cyst	_____	_____
Pregnancy	_____	_____
URI	_____	_____

Document 6

PATIENT INFORMATION SHEET

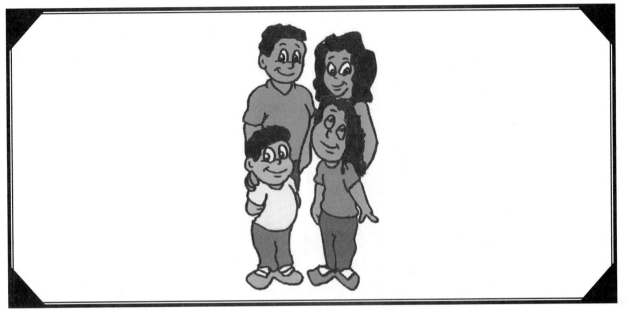

INSURED'S INFORMATION

Patient ID: ___POG5508-008___   Assigned Provider: _____   Birth date: *Aug. 18, 1962*

Name: (Last, First, Middle) ___O'Gen. Pat N..___   Sex: ___*Female*___

Address: (Inc City, State, Zip) *621 Cayhill Ave., Colter, CO 81222*

Home Phone: *(970) 555-3311*   Marital Status: *Single*   Social Security #: *333-33-3333*

Employer Name: ___*White Corporation*___   Work Phone: *(970) 555-1234 x591*

Employer Address: *1234 Whitaker Lane, Colter, CO 81250*

Employment Status: ___*Full-time*___   Referred by: _____

Allergies/Medical conditions: _____

Primary Ins Name: *Winter Insurance Co.*   Address: *9763 Western Way, Whittier, CO 82963*

ID #: *333-11-Whi*   Plan #/Name: *White Corp.*   Policy Holder Name: *Pat O'Gen*

Secondary Ins Name: ___*N/A*___   Address: _____

ID #: _____   Plan #/Name: _____   Policy Holder Name: _____

SPOUSE'S INFORMATION

Patient ID: ___COG5509-009___   Assigned Provider: _____   Birth date: *Nov. 12, 1964*

Name: (Last, First, Middle) ___O'Gen, Carson___   Sex: ___*Male*___

Social Security #: ___*331-32-3334*___   Employment Status: _____

Employer Name: *Self Employed*   Work Phone: _____

Employer Address: ___*621 Cayhill Ave., Colter, CO 81222*___

Allergies/Medical conditions: _____

Primary Ins Name: *Winter Insurance Co.*   Address: *9763 Western Way, Whittier, CO 82963*

ID #: *333-11-Whi*   Plan #/Name: *White Corp.*   Policy Holder Name: *Pat O'Gen*

Secondary Ins Name: ___*N/A*___   Address: _____

ID #: _____   Plan #/Name: _____   Policy Holder Name: _____

CHILD #1

Patient ID: __COG5510-010__   Assigned Provider: _____   Birth date: _Feb. 17, 1985_

Name of Minor Child: __O'Gen, Cass N.__   Social Security #: _303-17-1980_

Sex: _Female_   Marital Status: __Single__   Relationship to Insured: _Daughter_

Allergies/Medical conditions: _____

Primary Ins Name: _Winter Insurance Co.__   Primary Insured: __Mother__

Secondary Ins Name: __N/A__   Secondary Insured: _____

CHILD #2

Patient ID: __OOG5511-011__   Assigned Provider: _____   Birth date: _Feb. 11, 1995_

Name of Minor Child: __O'Gen, Ox__   Social Security #: _198-90-2114_

Sex: _Male_   Marital Status: __Single__   Relationship to Insured: _Son_

Allergies/Medical conditions: _____

Primary Ins Name: _Winter Insurance Co.__   Primary Insured: __Mother__

Secondary Ins Name: __N/A__   Secondary Insured: _____

CHILD #3

Patient ID: _____   Assigned Provider: _____   Birth date: _____

Name of Minor Child: _____   Social Security #: _____

Sex: _____   Marital Status: _____   Relationship to Insured: _____

Allergies/Medical conditions: _____

Primary Ins Name: _____   Primary Insured: _____

Secondary Ins Name: _____   Secondary Insured: _____

EMERGENCY CONTACT

Name: __C. R. Y. O'Gen__   Home Phone: _(970) 555- 4139_   Other Phone: _(970) 555-3406_

Address: (Inc City, State, Zip) __6548 Outofair Ave. Apt# A1,3 Colter, CO 81222__

ACKNOWLEDGMENT AND AUTHORITY FOR TREATMENT AND PAYMENT

_PO_   I consent to treatment as necessary or desirable to the care of the patient named above, including but not restricted to whatever drugs, medicine, performance of operations and conduct of laboratory, x-ray, or other studies that may be used by the attending doctor, his/her nurse or qualified designate:

_PO_   I also acknowledge full responsibility for the payment of such services and agree to pay for them upon demand, in full, AT THE TIME OF SERVICE. If the physician must use a collection agency/attorney or court to collect its charges, then I will pay reasonable attorney fees and costs incurred in collecting same, regardless of insurance coverage.

_PO_   I hereby authorize payment directly to Consolidated Health Services of the medical expense benefits otherwise payable to me but not to exceed my indebtedness to said physician on account of the enclosed charge.

_PO_   I hereby authorize any medical practitioner, medical or medically related facility, insurance or reinsuring company, consumer reporting agency, or employer having information with respect to any physical or mental condition and/or treatment of me or my minor children and any other non-medical information of me and my minor children to give to the group policy holder, my employer, or its legal representative, any and all such information.

_PO_   I understand the information obtained by the use of the Authorization will be used to determine eligibility for insurance, and eligibility for benefits under any existing policy. Any information obtained will not be released by/to any organization EXCEPT to the group policyholder, my employer, reinsuring companies, the Medical Information Bureau, Inc., or other persons or organizations performing business or legal services in connection with my application, claim, or as may be otherwise lawfully required or as I may further authorize.

_PO_   I further agree that a photographic copy of this Authorization shall be valid as the original. This Authorization shall be valid for one year from the date shown below.

Signature of Insured: __Pat N. O'Gen__   Date: __Jan. 14, 20XX__

Signature of Spouse: _____   Date: _____

PATIENT INFORMATION SHEET

INSURED'S INFORMATION

Patient ID: _CPE5512-012_   Assigned Provider: _____   Birth date: _Mar. 12, 1975_

Name: (Last, First, Middle) _Pendent, Codie_   Sex: _Female_

Address: (Inc City, State, Zip) _1111 E. Dunphy Drive, Colter, CO 81222_

Home Phone: _(970) 555-1965_   Marital Status: _Married_   Social Security #: _444-44-3985_

Employer Name: _Red Enterprises_   Work Phone: _(970) 555-0863_

Employer Address: _7677 Royal Road, Colter, CO 81293_

Employment Status: _Full-time_   Referred by: _PPO List_

Allergies/Medical conditions: _____

Primary Ins Name: _Rover Insurers, Inc._   Address: _5931 Rolling Road, Ronson, CO 81369_

ID #: _444-44-3985_   Plan #/Name: _41935Red_   Policy Holder Name: _Codie Pendent_

Secondary Ins Name: _N/A_   Address: _____

ID #: _____   Plan #/Name: _____   Policy Holder Name: _____

SPOUSE'S INFORMATION

Patient ID: _APE5513-013_   Assigned Provider: _____   Birth date: _May 15, 1973_

Name: (Last, First, Middle) _Pendent, Andy_   Sex: _Male_

Social Security #: _415-19-0563_   Employment Status: _Laid Off_

Employer Name: _KDDD Radio Station_   Work Phone: _____

Employer Address: _____

Allergies/Medical conditions: _____

Primary Ins Name: _See Wife_   Address: _____

ID #: _____   Plan #/Name: _____   Policy Holder Name: _____

Secondary Ins Name: _N/A_   Address: _____

ID #: _____   Plan #/Name: _____   Policy Holder Name: _____

CHILD #1

Patient ID: ___DPE5514-014___   Assigned Provider: _____   Birth date: _Apr. 12, 1998_

Name of Minor Child: _Pendent, Dee_____   Social Security #: _444-01-9912_____

Sex: _Female_____   Marital Status: ___Single_____   Relationship to Insured: _Daughter_____

Allergies/Medical conditions: _____

Primary Ins Name: _Rover Insurers, Inc._____   Primary Insured: __Mother_____

Secondary Ins Name: ___N/A_____   Secondary Insured: _____

CHILD #2

Patient ID: _____   Assigned Provider: _____   Birth date: _____

Name of Minor Child: _____   Social Security #: _____

Sex: _____   Marital Status: _____   Relationship to Insured: _____

Allergies/Medical conditions: _____

Primary Ins Name: _____   Primary Insured: _____

Secondary Ins Name: _____   Secondary Insured: _____

CHILD #3

Patient ID: _____   Assigned Provider: _____   Birth date: _____

Name of Minor Child: _____   Social Security #: _____

Sex: _____   Marital Status: _____   Relationship to Insured: _____

Allergies/Medical conditions: _____

Primary Ins Name: _____   Primary Insured: _____

Secondary Ins Name: _____   Secondary Insured: _____

EMERGENCY CONTACT

Name: _N. Abor_____   Home Phone: _(970) 555- 6095_____   Other Phone: _(970) 555- 3569_____

Address: (Inc City, State, Zip)___6518 N. Dunphy Drive Colter, CO 81222_____

ACKNOWLEDGMENT AND AUTHORITY FOR TREATMENT AND PAYMENT

___CD___ I consent to treatment as necessary or desirable to the care of the patient named above, including but not restricted to whatever drugs, medicine, performance of operations and conduct of laboratory, x-ray, or other studies that may be used by the attending doctor, his/her nurse or qualified designate:

___CD___ I also acknowledge full responsibility for the payment of such services and agree to pay for them upon demand, in full, AT THE TIME OF SERVICE. If the physician must use a collection agency/attorney or court to collect its charges, then I will pay reasonable attorney fees and costs incurred in collecting same, regardless of insurance coverage.

___CD___ I hereby authorize payment directly to Consolidated Health Services of the medical expense benefits otherwise payable to me but not to exceed my indebtedness to said physician on account of the enclosed charge.

___CD___ I hereby authorize any medical practitioner, medical or medically related facility, insurance or reinsuring company, consumer reporting agency, or employer having information with respect to any physical or mental condition and/or treatment of me or my minor children and any other non-medical information of me and my minor children to give to the group policy holder, my employer, or its legal representative, any and all such information.

___CD___ I understand the information obtained by the use of the Authorization will be used to determine eligibility for insurance, and eligibility for benefits under any existing policy. Any information obtained will not be released by/to any organization EXCEPT to the group policyholder, my employer, reinsuring companies, the Medical Information Bureau, Inc., or other persons or organizations performing business or legal services in connection with my application, claim, or as may be otherwise lawfully required or as I may further authorize.

___CD___ I further agree that a photographic copy of this Authorization shall be valid as the original. This Authorization shall be valid for one year from the date shown below.

Signature of Insured: __Codie Pendent_____   Date: __Jan. 1, 20XX_____

Signature of Spouse: _____   Date: _____

PROVIDER INFORMATION

7. **Provider:** Ben Dover, M.D., Gastroenterologist
   Address: 2468 Custom Blvd, Ste. 300, Colter, CO 81222
   Phone: (970) 555-6541
   License #: FF466646
   EIN: 40-2461234
   MCR UPIN: BWD006
   Provider Accepts Medicare Assignment   Rover Network Provider

8. **Provider:** Yu B. Sickman, M.D., G.P.
   Address: 1357 Castle Blvd, Ste. 501A, Colter, CO 81222
   Phone: (970) 555-3574
   License #: GG369741
   EIN: 40-3759772
   MCR UPIN: YBS001
   Provider Accepts Medicare Assignment

9. **Provider:** Butch M.N. Hackim, M.D., Surgeon
   Address: 1357 Castle Blvd, Ste. 510, Colter, CO 81222
   Phone: (970) 555-0954
   License #: HH852369
   EIN: 40-2159735
   MCR UPIN: BMH011
   Provider Accepts Medicare Assignment

10. **Provider:** Kent Cure, M.D., ER
    Address: 1357 Castle Blvd, Ste. 529, Colter, CO 81222
    Phone: (970) 555-5290
    License #: JJ963021
    EIN: 40-3445555
    MCR UPIN: KCC051
    Provider Accepts Medicare Assignment

11. **Provider:** Manny Kutz, M.D., Surgeon, Assistant
    Address: 1357 Castle Blvd, Ste. 506, Colter, CO 81222
    Phone: (970) 555-3001
    License #: KK987410
    EIN: 40-3159735
    MCR UPIN: MMK011
    Provider Accepts Medicare Assignment

12. **Provider:** Will Kutteroff, M.D., Surgeon
    Address: 1357 Castle Blvd, Ste. 507, Colter, CO 81222
    Phone: (970) 555-8652
    License #: MM654987
    EIN: 40-9999996
    MCR UPIN: WEK006
    Provider Accepts Medicare Assignment

PATIENT INFORMATION SHEET

INSURED'S INFORMATION

Patient ID: _JAT5515-015_   Assigned Provider: _____   Birth date: _Apr. 3, 1936_

Name: (Last, First, Middle) _Attricks, Jerry_   Sex: _Male_

Address: (Inc City, State, Zip) _Route 1 Box 83, Colter, CO 81235_

Home Phone: _(970) 555-5319_   Marital Status: _Married_   Social Security #: _555-23-5555_

Employer Name: _Blue Corporation_   Work Phone: _____

Employer Address: _9817 Bobcat Blvd., Bastion, CO 81319_

Employment Status: _Retired_   Referred by: _____

Allergies/Medical conditions: _____

Primary Ins Name: _Medicare_   Address: _1873 Montrose Ave., Minx, CO 82377_

ID #: _555-23-5555A_   Plan #/Name: _____   Policy Holder Name: _Jerry Attricks_

Secondary Ins Name: _N/A_   Address: _____

ID #: _____   Plan #/Name: _____   Policy Holder Name: _____

SPOUSE'S INFORMATION

Patient ID: _SAT5516-016_   Assigned Provider: _____   Birth date: _Mar. 12, 1938_

Name: (Last, First, Middle) _Attricks, Sherry_   Sex: _Female_

Social Security #: _515-51-5151_   Employment Status: _Full-time_

Employer Name: _Blue Corporation_   Work Phone: _(970) 555-9876_

Employer Address: _9817 Bobcat Blvd., Bastion, CO 81319_

Allergies/Medical conditions: _____

Primary Ins Name: _Ball Insurance Carriers_   Address: _3895 Bubble Blvd. Ste. 283, Boxwood, CO 85931_

ID #: _515-51-Blue_   Plan #/Name: _98135Blue_   Policy Holder Name: _Sherry Attricks_

Secondary Ins Name: _N/A_   Address: _____

ID #: _____   Plan #/Name: _____   Policy Holder Name: _____

CHILD #1

Patient ID: ___*PAT5517-017*___ Assigned Provider: _____ Birth date: *Jun. 28, 1985*

Name of Minor Child: ___*Attricks, Petey*___ Social Security #: *556-19-2879*

Sex: *Male*_____ Marital Status: ___*Single*___ Relationship to Insured: *Grandchild*_____

Allergies/Medical conditions: ___*FTS Colton Community College*___

Primary Ins Name: *Ball Insurance Carrier*_____ Primary Insured: ___*Grandmother*___

Secondary Ins Name: ___*N/A*___ Secondary Insured: _____

CHILD #2

Patient ID: _____ Assigned Provider: _____ Birth date:_____

Name of Minor Child: _____ Social Security #: _____

Sex: _____ Marital Status: _____ Relationship to Insured: _____

Allergies/Medical conditions: _____

Primary Ins Name: _____ Primary Insured: _____

Secondary Ins Name: _____ Secondary Insured: _____

CHILD #3

Patient ID: _____ Assigned Provider: _____ Birth date:_____

Name of Minor Child: _____ Social Security #: _____

Sex: _____ Marital Status: _____ Relationship to Insured: _____

Allergies/Medical conditions: _____

Primary Ins Name: _____ Primary Insured: _____

Secondary Ins Name: _____ Secondary Insured: _____

EMERGENCY CONTACT

Name: ___*Vy Agra*___ Home Phone: *(970) 555-5396* Other Phone: *(970) 555-0659*_____

Address: (Inc City, State, Zip)___*Route 2 Box 38, Colter, CO 81235*___

ACKNOWLEDGMENT AND AUTHORITY FOR TREATMENT AND PAYMENT

___*SA*___ I consent to treatment as necessary or desirable to the care of the patient named above, including but not restricted to whatever drugs, medicine, performance of operations and conduct of laboratory, x-ray, or other studies that may be used by the attending doctor, his/her nurse or qualified designate:

___*SA*___ I also acknowledge full responsibility for the payment of such services and agree to pay for them upon demand, in full, AT THE TIME OF SERVICE. If the physician must use a collection agency/attorney or court to collect its charges, then I will pay reasonable attorney fees and costs incurred in collecting same, regardless of insurance coverage.

___*SA*___ I hereby authorize payment directly to Consolidated Health Services of the medical expense benefits otherwise payable to me but not to exceed my indebtedness to said physician on account of the enclosed charge.

___*SA*___ I hereby authorize any medical practitioner, medical or medically related facility, insurance or reinsuring company, consumer reporting agency, or employer having information with respect to any physical or mental condition and/or treatment of me or my minor children and any other non-medical information of me and my minor children to give to the group policy holder, my employer, or its legal representative, any and all such information.

___*SA*___ I understand the information obtained by the use of the Authorization will be used to determine eligibility for insurance, and eligibility for benefits under any existing policy. Any information obtained will not be released by/to any organization EXCEPT to the group policyholder, my employer, reinsuring companies, the Medical Information Bureau, Inc., or other persons or organizations performing business or legal services in connection with my application, claim, or as may be otherwise lawfully required or as I may further authorize.

___*SA*___ I further agree that a photographic copy of this Authorization shall be valid as the original. This Authorization shall be valid for one year from the date shown below.

Signature of Insured: _____ Date: _____

Signature of Spouse: ___*Sherry Attricks*___ Date: ___*Jan. 14, 20XX*___

Appointment Calendar

DAY: _____Tuesday_____   DATE: _____January 22, 20XX_____

Time	Dr. Phil Goode	Dr. Yu B. Sickman	Dr. Allota Payne
8:00	CHS Hosp. Outpatient Dept.	Meeting	
8:15	↓	↓	
8:30	↓	↓	
8:45	↓	↓	
9:00	↓	Mal Adjusted	
9:15	↓	Sharon Needles	
9:30	↓	Anna Recksic	
9:45	↓	Di R. Rhea (10)/Mona Littlemore (5)	
10:00	↓		
10:15	↓	Wilma Leggrow-Bach	
10:30	↓	↓	
10:45	↓		
11:00	↓	Dennis Elbow (20)	
11:15	↓		
11:30	↓		
11:45	↓	Denise R. Wobbly	
12:00	↓	Lunch Mtg./Dr. Kauf	
12:15	↓	↓	
12:30	Lunch	↓	
12:45	↓	↓	
1:00	↓	↓	
1:15	↓	↓	
1:30	↓	Mary Mumps	
1:45	↓	Melissa Mumps	
2:00		Sam Manilla (25)	
2:15		↓	
2:30		Cher D. Virus (20)	
2:45			
3:00			
3:15			
3:30			
3:45			
4:00			
4:15			
4:30			
4:45			
5:00	Home	Home	
5:15	↓	↓	
5:30	↓	↓	
5:45	↓	↓	
6:00	↓	↓	

PATIENT INFORMATION SHEET

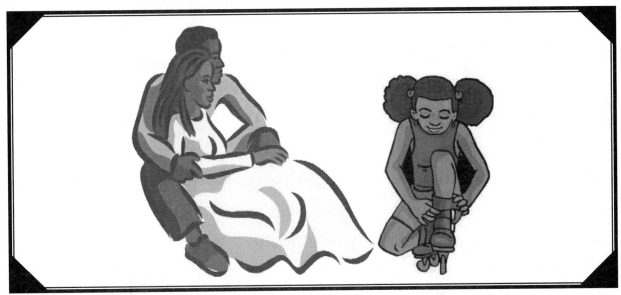

INSURED'S INFORMATION

Patient ID: ___GPO5518-018___ Assigned Provider: _____ Birth date: _Jun. 20, 1972_

Name: (Last, First, Middle) _Poole, Gene_ Sex: ___Male___

Address: (Inc City, State, Zip) _4738 Jessup Road, Jasper, CO 81335_

Home Phone: _(970) 555-1335_ Marital Status: _Common Law Marr_ Social Security #: _999-99-1985_

Employer Name: _White Corporation_ Work Phone: _(970) 555-1234 x631_

Employer Address: _1234 Whitaker Lane, Colter, CO 81250_

Employment Status: ___Full-time___ Referred by: ___Co-worker___

Allergies/Medical conditions: _____

Primary Ins Name: _Winter Insurance Co._ Address: _9763 Western Way, Whittier, CO 82963_

ID #: _999-99-Whi_ Plan #/Name: _White Corp._ Policy Holder Name: _Gene Poole_

Secondary Ins Name: ___N/A___ Address: _____

ID #: _____ Plan #/Name: _____ Policy Holder Name: _____

SPOUSE'S INFORMATION

Patient ID: ___JNE5519-019___ Assigned Provider: _____ Birth date: _Oct. 4, 1972_

Name: (Last, First, Middle) _Akenja-Nearing, Jeanette (she uses her maiden name)_ Sex: ___Female___

Social Security #: _919-99-1046_ Employment Status: ___Part-time___

Employer Name: _Jolly Jugglers Entertainment_ Work Phone: _(970) 555-6000_

Employer Address: ___5097 Justin Way, Jasper, CO 81355_

Allergies/Medical conditions: _____

Primary Ins Name: _See Gene Poole_ Address: _____

ID #: _____ Plan #/Name: _____ Policy Holder Name: _____

Secondary Ins Name: ___N/A___ Address: _____

ID #: _____ Plan #/Name: _____ Policy Holder Name: _____

CHILD #1

Patient ID: _CPO5520-020_   Assigned Provider: _____   Birth date: _Sep. 7, 1992_

Name of Minor Child: _Poole, Carla ("Car")_   Social Security #: _983-19-0907_

Sex: _Female_   Marital Status: _Single_   Relationship to Insured: _Daughter_

Allergies/Medical conditions: _____

Primary Ins Name: _Winter Insurance Co._   Primary Insured: _Mother_

Secondary Ins Name: _N/A_   Secondary Insured: _____

CHILD #2

Patient ID: _____   Assigned Provider: _____   Birth date: _____

Name of Minor Child: _____   Social Security #: _____

Sex: _____   Marital Status: _____   Relationship to Insured: _____

Allergies/Medical conditions: _____

Primary Ins Name: _____   Primary Insured: _____

Secondary Ins Name: _____   Secondary Insured: _____

CHILD #3

Patient ID: _____   Assigned Provider: _____   Birth date: _____

Name of Minor Child: _____   Social Security #: _____

Sex: _____   Marital Status: _____   Relationship to Insured: _____

Allergies/Medical conditions: _____

Primary Ins Name: _____   Primary Insured: _____

Secondary Ins Name: _____   Secondary Insured: _____

EMERGENCY CONTACT

Name: _Lotta Kids_   Home Phone: _(970) 555- 0301_   Other Phone: _(970) 555- 4488_

Address: (Inc City, State, Zip)   _4783 Childers Road, Jasper, CO 81335_

ACKNOWLEDGMENT AND AUTHORITY FOR TREATMENT AND PAYMENT

_GP_   I consent to treatment as necessary or desirable to the care of the patient named above, including but not restricted to whatever drugs, medicine, performance of operations and conduct of laboratory, x-ray, or other studies that may be used by the attending doctor, his/her nurse or qualified designate:

_GP_   I also acknowledge full responsibility for the payment of such services and agree to pay for them upon demand, in full, AT THE TIME OF SERVICE. If the physician must use a collection agency/attorney or court to collect its charges, then I will pay reasonable attorney fees and costs incurred in collecting same, regardless of insurance coverage.

_GP_   I hereby authorize payment directly to Consolidated Health Services of the medical expense benefits otherwise payable to me but not to exceed my indebtedness to said physician on account of the enclosed charge.

_GP_   I hereby authorize any medical practitioner, medical or medically related facility, insurance or reinsuring company, consumer reporting agency, or employer having information with respect to any physical or mental condition and/or treatment of me or my minor children and any other non-medical information of me and my minor children to give to the group policy holder, my employer, or its legal representative, any and all such information.

_GP_   I understand the information obtained by the use of the Authorization will be used to determine eligibility for insurance, and eligibility for benefits under any existing policy. Any information obtained will not be released by/to any organization EXCEPT to the group policyholder, my employer, reinsuring companies, the Medical Information Bureau, Inc., or other persons or organizations performing business or legal services in connection with my application, claim, or as may be otherwise lawfully required or as I may further authorize.

_GP_   I further agree that a photographic copy of this Authorization shall be valid as the original. This Authorization shall be valid for one year from the date shown below.

Signature of Insured: _Gene Poole_   Date: _Jan. 8, 20XX_

Signature of Spouse: _____   Date: _____

PATIENT INFORMATION SHEET

INSURED'S INFORMATION

Patient ID: ___*RAL5521-021*___ Assigned Provider: _____ Birth date: *Nov. 25, 1960*

Name: (Last, First, Middle) __*Allity, Ray*__ Sex: ___*Male*___

Address: (Inc City, State, Zip) *426 Kirby Street, Colton, CO 81223*

Home Phone: *(970) 555-7210* Marital Status: *Divorced* Social Security #: *011-11-0011*

Employer Name: __*Red Enterprises*__ Work Phone: *(970) 555-0863*

Employer Address: *7677 Royal Road, Colter, CO 81293*

Employment Status: ___*Full-time*___ Referred by: ___*PPO List*___

Allergies/Medical conditions: _____

Primary Ins Name: *Rover Insurers, Inc.* Address: *5931 Rolling Road, Ronson, CO 81369*

ID #: *011-11-0011* Plan #/Name: *41935Red* Policy Holder Name: *Ray Allity*

Secondary Ins Name: ___*N/A*___ Address: _____

ID #: _____ Plan #/Name: _____ Policy Holder Name: _____

SPOUSE'S INFORMATION

Patient ID: _____ Assigned Provider: _____ Birth date: _____

Name: (Last, First, Middle) __*N/A*__ Sex: _____

Social Security #: _____ Employment Status: _____

Employer Name: _____ Work Phone: _____

Employer Address: _____

Allergies/Medical conditions: _____

Primary Ins Name: _____ Address: _____

ID #: _____ Plan #/Name: _____ Policy Holder Name: _____

Secondary Ins Name: _____ Address: _____

ID #: _____ Plan #/Name: _____ Policy Holder Name: _____

CHILD #1

Patient ID: _RAL5522-022_   Assigned Provider: _____   Birth date: _Nov. 25, 1990_

Name of Minor Child: _Allity, Rhea_   Social Security #: _110-41-8921_

Sex: _Female_   Marital Status: _Single_   Relationship to Insured: _Daughter_

Allergies/Medical conditions: _____

Primary Ins Name: _Rover Insurer, Inc._   Primary Insured: _Father_

Secondary Ins Name: _N/A_   Secondary Insured: _____

CHILD #2

Patient ID: _MAL5523-023_   Assigned Provider: _____   Birth date: _Mar. 10, 1991_

Name of Minor Child: _Allity, Mort_   Social Security #: _113-10-9783_

Sex: _Male_   Marital Status: _Single_   Relationship to Insured: _Son_

Allergies/Medical conditions: _____

Primary Ins Name: _Rover Insurers, Inc._   Primary Insured: _Father_

Secondary Ins Name: _N/A_   Secondary Insured: _____

CHILD #3

Patient ID: _____   Assigned Provider: _____   Birth date: _____

Name of Minor Child: _____   Social Security #: _____

Sex: _____   Marital Status: _____   Relationship to Insured: _____

Allergies/Medical conditions: _____

Primary Ins Name: _____   Primary Insured: _____

Secondary Ins Name: _____   Secondary Insured: _____

EMERGENCY CONTACT

Name: _Mort Tician_   Home Phone: _(970) 555-2169_   Other Phone: _(970) 555-6560_

Address: (Inc City, State, Zip)   _9568 Littlelight Rd,. Colton, CO 81223_

ACKNOWLEDGMENT AND AUTHORITY FOR TREATMENT AND PAYMENT

_RA_   I consent to treatment as necessary or desirable to the care of the patient named above, including but not restricted to whatever drugs, medicine, performance of operations and conduct of laboratory, x-ray, or other studies that may be used by the attending doctor, his/her nurse or qualified designate:

_RA_   I also acknowledge full responsibility for the payment of such services and agree to pay for them upon demand, in full, AT THE TIME OF SERVICE. If the physician must use a collection agency/attorney or court to collect its charges, then I will pay reasonable attorney fees and costs incurred in collecting same, regardless of insurance coverage.

_RA_   I hereby authorize payment directly to Consolidated Health Services of the medical expense benefits otherwise payable to me but not to exceed my indebtedness to said physician on account of the enclosed charge.

_RA_   I hereby authorize any medical practitioner, medical or medically related facility, insurance or reinsuring company, consumer reporting agency, or employer having information with respect to any physical or mental condition and/or treatment of me or my minor children and any other non-medical information of me and my minor children to give to the group policy holder, my employer, or its legal representative, any and all such information.

_RA_   I understand the information obtained by the use of the Authorization will be used to determine eligibility for insurance, and eligibility for benefits under any existing policy. Any information obtained will not be released by/to any organization EXCEPT to the group policyholder, my employer, reinsuring companies, the Medical Information Bureau, Inc., or other persons or organizations performing business or legal services in connection with my application, claim, or as may be otherwise lawfully required or as I may further authorize.

_RA_   I further agree that a photographic copy of this Authorization shall be valid as the original. This Authorization shall be valid for one year from the date shown below.

Signature of Insured: _Ray Allity_   Date: _Jan. 4, 20XX_

Signature of Spouse: _____   Date: _____

PATIENT INFORMATION SHEET

INSURED'S INFORMATION

Patient ID: ___AKN5524-024___ Assigned Provider: _____ Birth date: _Jul. 27, 1971_

Name: (Last, First, Middle) _____Knose, Al Weighs_____ Sex: ___Male___

Address: (Inc City, State, Zip) _56789 Hamer Lane, Colter, CO 81222_

Home Phone: _(970) 555-5678_ Marital Status: _Married_ Social Security #: _881-11-8888_

Employer Name: _Self-Employed_ Work Phone:_____

Employer Address: _See Above_

Employment Status: ___Full-time___ Referred by: _____

Allergies/Medical conditions: _____

Primary Ins Name: ___N/A___ Address:_____

ID #:_____ Plan #/Name: _____ Policy Holder Name:_____

Secondary Ins Name: ___N/A___ Address: _____

ID #: _____ Plan #/Name: _____ Policy Holder Name: _____

SPOUSE'S INFORMATION

Patient ID: ___IKN5525-025___ Assigned Provider: _____ Birth date: _Jan. 7, 1975_

Name: (Last, First, Middle) __Knose, Ima__ Sex: ___Female___

Social Security #: _919-88-8598_ Employment Status: ___Homemaker___

Employer Name: _Self-employed_ Work Phone:_____

Employer Address: _____

Allergies/Medical conditions: _____

Primary Ins Name: ___N/A___ Address: _____

ID #:_____ Plan #/Name: _____ Policy Holder Name:_____

Secondary Ins Name: ___N/A___ Address: _____

ID #: _____ Plan #/Name: _____ Policy Holder Name: _____

CHILD #1

Patient ID: ___RKN5526-026___ Assigned Provider: _____ Birth date: *Oct. 17, 1997*

Name of Minor Child: ___Knose, Ron E.___ Social Security #: *810-17-8818*

Sex: *Male* _____ Marital Status: ___Single___ Relationship to Insured: *Son*

Allergies/Medical conditions: ___Cerebral Palsy___

Primary Ins Name: *None* _____ Primary Insured: _____

Secondary Ins Name: ___N/A___ Secondary Insured: _____

CHILD #2

Patient ID: ___AKN5527-027___ Assigned Provider: _____ Birth date: *Jun. 22, 2000*

Name of Minor Child: ___Knose Beane Andy___ Social Security #: *810-22-9588*

Sex: *Male* _____ Marital Status: ___Single___ Relationship to Insured: *Son*

Allergies/Medical conditions: _____

Primary Ins Name: *None* _____ Primary Insured: _____

Secondary Ins Name: ___N/A___ Secondary Insured: _____

CHILD #3

Patient ID: _____ Assigned Provider: _____ Birth date_____

Name of Minor Child: _____ Social Security #: _____

Sex: _____ Marital Status: _____ Relationship to Insured: _____

Allergies/Medical conditions: _____

Primary Ins Name: _____ Primary Insured: _____

Secondary Ins Name: _____ Secondary Insured: _____

EMERGENCY CONTACT

Name: ___Noel Itall___ Home Phone: *(970) 555-2189* Other Phone: *(970) 555-3630*

Address: (Inc City, State, Zip)___56432 Library Lane, Colter, CO 81222___

ACKNOWLEDGMENT AND AUTHORITY FOR TREATMENT AND PAYMENT

___IK___   I consent to treatment as necessary or desirable to the care of the patient named above, including but not restricted to whatever drugs, medicine, performance of operations and conduct of laboratory, x-ray, or other studies that may be used by the attending doctor, his/her nurse or qualified designate:

___IK___   I also acknowledge full responsibility for the payment of such services and agree to pay for them upon demand, in full, AT THE TIME OF SERVICE. If the physician must use a collection agency/attorney or court to collect its charges, then I will pay reasonable attorney fees and costs incurred in collecting same, regardless of insurance coverage.

___IK___   I hereby authorize payment directly to Consolidated Health Services of the medical expense benefits otherwise payable to me but not to exceed my indebtedness to said physician on account of the enclosed charge.

___IK___   I hereby authorize any medical practitioner, medical or medically related facility, insurance or reinsuring company, consumer reporting agency, or employer having information with respect to any physical or mental condition and/or treatment of me or my minor children and any other non-medical information of me and my minor children to give to the group policy holder, my employer, or its legal representative, any and all such information.

___IK___   I understand the information obtained by the use of the Authorization will be used to determine eligibility for insurance, and eligibility for benefits under any existing policy. Any information obtained will not be released by/to any organization EXCEPT to the group policyholder, my employer, reinsuring companies, the Medical Information Bureau, Inc., or other persons or organizations performing business or legal services in connection with my application, claim, or as may be otherwise lawfully required or as I may further authorize.

___IK___   I further agree that a photographic copy of this Authorization shall be valid as the original. This Authorization shall be valid for one year from the date shown below.

Signature of Insured: _____ Date: _____

Signature of Spouse: ___Ima Knose___ Date: ___Jan. 14, 20XX___

Document 14

PATIENT INFORMATION SHEET

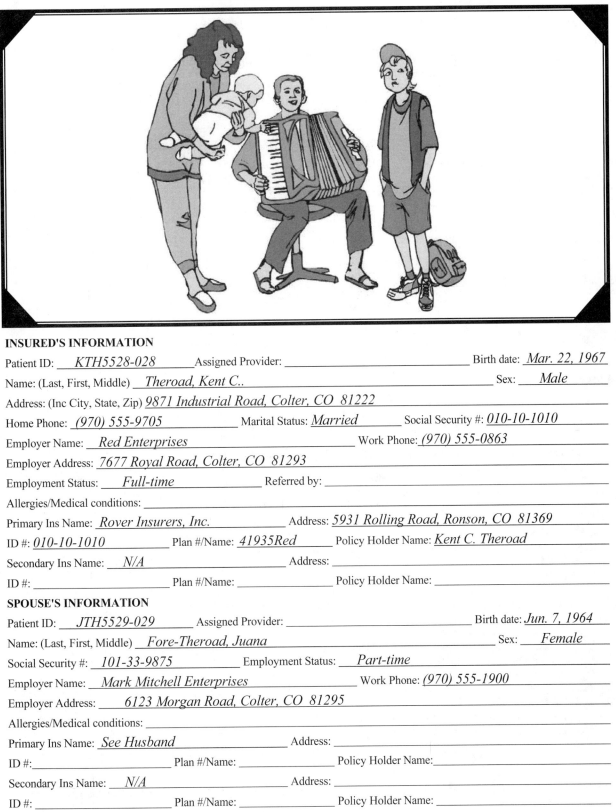

INSURED'S INFORMATION

Patient ID: __KTH5528-028__ Assigned Provider: _____ Birth date: _Mar. 22, 1967_

Name: (Last, First, Middle) _Theroad, Kent C.._ Sex: _Male_

Address: (Inc City, State, Zip) _9871 Industrial Road, Colter, CO 81222_

Home Phone: _(970) 555-9705_ Marital Status: _Married_ Social Security #: _010-10-1010_

Employer Name: _Red Enterprises_ Work Phone: _(970) 555-0863_

Employer Address: _7677 Royal Road, Colter, CO 81293_

Employment Status: _Full-time_ Referred by: _____

Allergies/Medical conditions: _____

Primary Ins Name: _Rover Insurers, Inc._ Address: _5931 Rolling Road, Ronson, CO 81369_

ID #: _010-10-1010_ Plan #/Name: _41935Red_ Policy Holder Name: _Kent C. Theroad_

Secondary Ins Name: _N/A_ Address: _____

ID #: _____ Plan #/Name: _____ Policy Holder Name: _____

SPOUSE'S INFORMATION

Patient ID: __JTH5529-029__ Assigned Provider: _____ Birth date: _Jun. 7, 1964_

Name: (Last, First, Middle) _Fore-Theroad, Juana_ Sex: _Female_

Social Security #: _101-33-9875_ Employment Status: _Part-time_

Employer Name: _Mark Mitchell Enterprises_ Work Phone: _(970) 555-1900_

Employer Address: _6123 Morgan Road, Colter, CO 81295_

Allergies/Medical conditions: _____

Primary Ins Name: _See Husband_ Address: _____

ID #: _____ Plan #/Name: _____ Policy Holder Name: _____

Secondary Ins Name: _N/A_ Address: _____

ID #: _____ Plan #/Name: _____ Policy Holder Name: _____

CHILD #1

Patient ID: _____ITH5530-030_____   Assigned Provider: _____   Birth date: *Sep. 2, 1991*

Name of Minor Child: _____*Theroad, Ian N.*_____   Social Security #: _*101-02-1982*_

Sex: *Male*_____   Marital Status: _____*Single*_____   Relationship to Insured: *Son*_____

Allergies/Medical conditions: _____

Primary Ins Name: *Rover Insurers, Inc.*_____   Primary Insured: _*Father*_____

Secondary Ins Name: _*N/A*_____   Secondary Insured: _____

CHILD #2

Patient ID: _____DTH5531-031_____   Assigned Provider: _____   Birth date: *Jul. 1, 2003*

Name of Minor Child: _____*Theroad, Donette*_____   Social Security #: _*101-71-7989*_

Sex: *Female*_____   Marital Status: _____*Single*_____   Relationship to Insured: *Daughter*_____

Allergies/Medical conditions: _____

Primary Ins Name: *Rover Insurers, Inc.*_____   Primary Insured: _*Father*_____

Secondary Ins Name: _*N/A*_____   Secondary Insured: _____

CHILD #3

Patient ID: _____   Assigned Provider: _____   Birth date: _____

Name of Minor Child: _____   Social Security #: _____

Sex: _____   Marital Status: _____   Relationship to Insured: _____

Allergies/Medical conditions: _____

Primary Ins Name: _____   Primary Insured: _____

Secondary Ins Name: _____   Secondary Insured: _____

EMERGENCY CONTACT

Name: _*Ima N. Theroad*_____   Home Phone: *(970) 555- 5132*_____   Other Phone: *(970) 555- 4334*_____

Address: (Inc City, State, Zip)_____*666 Roadahead Colter, CO 81222*_____

ACKNOWLEDGMENT AND AUTHORITY FOR TREATMENT AND PAYMENT

KCT I consent to treatment as necessary or desirable to the care of the patient named above, including but not restricted to whatever drugs, medicine, performance of operations and conduct of laboratory, x-ray, or other studies that may be used by the attending doctor, his/her nurse or qualified designate:

KCT I also acknowledge full responsibility for the payment of such services and agree to pay for them upon demand, in full, AT THE TIME OF SERVICE. If the physician must use a collection agency/attorney or court to collect its charges, then I will pay reasonable attorney fees and costs incurred in collecting same, regardless of insurance coverage.

KCT I hereby authorize payment directly to Consolidated Health Services of the medical expense benefits otherwise payable to me but not to exceed my indebtedness to said physician on account of the enclosed charge.

KCT I hereby authorize any medical practitioner, medical or medically related facility, insurance or reinsuring company, consumer reporting agency, or employer having information with respect to any physical or mental condition and/or treatment of me or my minor children and any other non-medical information of me and my minor children to give to the group policy holder, my employer, or its legal representative, any and all such information.

KCT I understand the information obtained by the use of the Authorization will be used to determine eligibility for insurance, and eligibility for benefits under any existing policy. Any information obtained will not be released by/to any organization EXCEPT to the group policyholder, my employer, reinsuring companies, the Medical Information Bureau, Inc., or other persons or organizations performing business or legal services in connection with my application, claim, or as may be otherwise lawfully required or as I may further authorize.

KCT I further agree that a photographic copy of this Authorization shall be valid as the original. This Authorization shall be valid for one year from the date shown below.

Signature of Insured: _____*Kent C. Theroad*_____   Date: _*Jan. 14, 20XX*_____

Signature of Spouse: _____   Date: _____

PATIENT INFORMATION SHEET

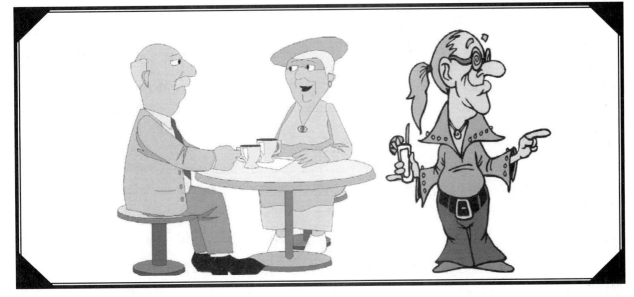

INSURED'S INFORMATION

Patient ID: ___HCU5532-032___   Assigned Provider: _____   Birth date: _Nov. 9, 1924_

Name: (Last, First, Middle) _Cupp, Hick_ _____   Sex: ___Male___

Address: (Inc City, State, Zip) _4231 Flame Blvd., Fulton, CO 81250_ _____

Home Phone: _(970) 555-8371_ _____   Marital Status: _Married_   Social Security #: _611-09-6666_

Employer Name: _White Corporation_ _____   Work Phone: _(970) 555-1234_ _____

Employer Address: _1234 Whitaker Lane, Colter, CO 81250_ _____

Employment Status: ___Retired___   Referred by: ___Avery Niceman_ _____

Allergies/Medical conditions: _____

Primary Ins Name: _Medicare_ _____   Address: _1873 Montrose Ave., Minx, CO 82377_ _____

ID #: _611-09-6666A_   Plan #/Name: _____   Policy Holder Name: _Hick Cup_

Secondary Ins Name: ___Winter Insurance Co._   Address: _9763 Western Way, Whittier, CO 82963_ _____

ID #: _611-09-Whi_   Plan #/Name: _Medigap_   Policy Holder Name: _Hick Cupp_ _____

SPOUSE'S INFORMATION

Patient ID: ___DCU5533-033___   Assigned Provider: _____   Birth date: _Oct. 8, 1929_

Name: (Last, First, Middle) _Cupp, Dee D._ _____   Sex: ___Female___

Social Security #: ___616-61-6161___   Employment Status: ___Retired___ _____

Employer Name: ___Homemaker___ _____   Work Phone: _____

Employer Address: _____

Allergies/Medical conditions: _____

Primary Ins Name: _Medicare_ _____   Address: _1873 Montrose Ave. Minx, CO 82377_ _____

ID #: _616-61-6161A_   Plan #/Name: _____   Policy Holder Name: _Dee D. Cupp_ _____

Secondary Ins Name: ___Winter Insurance Co._   Address: _9763 Western Way, Whittier, CO 82377_

ID #: _611-09Whi_   Plan #/Name: _Medigap_   Policy Holder Name: _Hick Cupp_ _____

CHILD #1

Patient ID: ___PCU5534-034___   Assigned Provider: _____   Birth date: _Dec. 8, 1953_

Name of Minor Child: ___Cupp, Phillip D.___   Social Security #: _626-62-6262_

Sex: _Male_   Marital Status: ___Single___   Relationship to Insured: _Self_

Allergies/Medical conditions: ___ESRD diagnosed 8/5/01 Dialysis begun 9/3/01___

Primary Ins Name: _Winter Insurance Co._   Address: _9763 Western Way, Whittier CO 82963_

ID #: _626-62-Whi_   Plan #/Name: _White Corp_   Policy Holder Name: _Phillip D. Cupp_

Secondary Ins Name: ___N/A___   Address:_____

ID #: _626-62-6262HDA_   Plan #/Name: _____   Policy Holder Name: _Phillip D. Cupp_

CHILD #2

Patient ID: _____   Assigned Provider: _____   Birth date:_____

Name of Minor Child: _____   Social Security #: _____

Sex: _____   Marital Status: _____   Relationship to Insured: _____

Allergies/Medical conditions: _____

Primary Ins Name: _____   Address: _____

ID #: _____   Plan #/Name: _____   Policy Holder Name: _____

Secondary Ins Name: _____   Address: _____

ID #: _____   Plan #/Name: _____   Policy Holder Name: _____

EMERGENCY CONTACT

Name: ___Dixie Cupp___   Home Phone: _(970) 555-7813_   Other Phone: _(970) 555-8000_

Address: (Inc City, State, Zip)___40333 177th St., Fulton, CO 81250___

ACKNOWLEDGMENT AND AUTHORITY FOR TREATMENT AND PAYMENT

___HC___   I consent to treatment as necessary or desirable to the care of the patient named above, including but not restricted to whatever drugs, medicine, performance of operations and conduct of laboratory, x-ray, or other studies that may be used by the attending doctor, his/her nurse or qualified designate:

___HC___   I also acknowledge full responsibility for the payment of such services and agree to pay for them upon demand, in full, AT THE TIME OF SERVICE. If the physician must use a collection agency/attorney or court to collect its charges, then I will pay reasonable attorney fees and costs incurred in collecting same, regardless of insurance coverage.

___HC___   I hereby authorize payment directly to Consolidated Health Services of the medical expense benefits otherwise payable to me but not to exceed my indebtedness to said physician on account of the enclosed charge.

___HC___   I hereby authorize any medical practitioner, medical or medically related facility, insurance or reinsuring company, consumer reporting agency, or employer having information with respect to any physical or mental condition and/or treatment of me or my minor children and any other non-medical information of me and my minor children to give to the group policy holder, my employer, or its legal representative, any and all such information.

___HC___   I understand the information obtained by the use of the Authorization will be used to determine eligibility for insurance, and eligibility for benefits under any existing policy. Any information obtained will not be released by/to any organization EXCEPT to the group policyholder, my employer, reinsuring companies, the Medical Information Bureau, Inc., or other persons or organizations performing business or legal services in connection with my application, claim, or as may be otherwise lawfully required or as I may further authorize.

___HC___   I further agree that a photographic copy of this Authorization shall be valid as the original. This Authorization shall be valid for one year from the date shown below.

Signature of Insured: ___Hick Cupp___   Date: _Jan. 1, 20XX_

Signature of Spouse: ___Dee D. Cupp___   Date: _Jan. 1, 20XX_

Phillip D. Cupp   *January 3, 20XX*

Phillip works full-time for White Corp. as an office assistant.

BALL INSURANCE CARRIERS

(800) 555-5432

3895 Bubble Blvd. Ste. 283, Boxwood, CO 85926

(970) 555-5432

Effective 09/1/93

PLAN: **Blue Corporation Contract**

INSURANCE CONTACT:__**Betty Bell**_____   PHONE NUMBER:__**(970) 555-5433**__

ELIGIBILITY

EMPLOYEE: Must work a minimum of 30 hours per week. Is eligible for coverage the first of the month following three consecutive months of continuous employment.

DEPENDENTS: Eligible for coverage from birth to age 19, or to age 23 if a full-time student or handicapped prior to 19/23 (proof of disability must be furnished within 31 days after dependent reaches limiting age). Not eligible as a dependent if eligible as an employee. Unmarried natural children, legally adopted/foster children included (also legal guardianship). If both parents are covered by the plan, children may be covered by one employee only.

EFFECTIVE DATE

EMPLOYEE: If written application is made prior to eligibility date, coverage becomes effective the first of the month following three months of continuous employment.

DEPENDENTS: The date acquired by the covered employee becomes the effective date if written application is made within 31 days of eligibility date. If confined in a hospital on date of eligibility, coverage will not start until the first of the month following the date the confinement ends. Newborns are auto-matically covered for the first 30 days following birth. Coverage will be terminated after 30 days unless written application for coverage is submitted by the employee within 31 days of birth.

TERMINATION OF COVERAGE

EMPLOYEE: Coverage terminates the last day of the month following termination of employment, or when the employee ceases to qualify as an eligible employee, or following request for termination of coverage.

DEPENDENTS: Coverage terminates the date the employee's coverage terminates or the last day of the month during which the dependent no longer qualifies as an eligible dependent.

BASIC BENEFITS

PRE-ADMISSION TESTING - Out-patient diagnostic tests done prior to inpatient admit; paid at 100% of UCR.

SUPPLEMENTAL ACCIDENT EXPENSE - 100% of the first $300.00 for services within 90 days of accident.

INPATIENT HOSPITAL EXPENSE

DEDUCTIBLE: $50.

ROOM AND BOARD: Up to semi-private room charge. ICU up to $600.00 per day.

MISCELLANEOUS FEES: Unlimited.

MAXIMUM PERIOD: 10 days per period of disability.

SURGERY

CONVERSION FACTOR: $8.50.

CALENDAR YEAR MAXIMUM: $1,600 per person.

REMARKS: Voluntary sterilizations covered.

ASSISTANT SURGERY

CONVERSION FACTOR: $8.50.

CALENDAR YEAR MAXIMUM ALLOWANCE: $320 per person. Maximum of 20% of surgeon's allowance or billed charge, whichever is less.

REMARKS: Voluntary sterilizations covered for women only.

IN-HOSPITAL PHYSICIANS

DAILY MAXIMUM: $21 for the first day; $8 per day thereafter.

MAXIMUM PERIOD: Ten days per period of disability.

REMARKS: Only one doctor can be paid per day.

ANESTHESIA

CONVERSION FACTOR: $7.50.

CALENDAR YEAR MAXIMUM: $300 per person.

REMARKS: Voluntary sterilizations covered.

OUTPATIENT PHYSICIANS VISITS

CONVERSION FACTOR: $7.50.

CALENDAR YEAR MAXIMUM: $300 per person.

REMARKS: Chiropractors, M.D.s, DOs and acupuncturists allowed. Mental and Nervous treatment not covered.

X-RAY AND LABORATORY

CONVERSION FACTOR: $7.
CALENDAR YEAR MAXIMUM: $200 per person.
REMARKS: Professional component covered at 40% of UCR for procedure. Routine procedures are not covered.

MAJOR MEDICAL EXPENSES

INDIVIDUAL CALENDAR YEAR DEDUCTIBLE: $125; three month carryover provision.
FAMILY MAXIMUM DEDUCTIBLE: Two family members must satisfy their individual calendar year deductible in order to satisfy the family deductible.
STANDARD COINSURANCE: 80%.
COINSURANCE LIMIT: $400 out-of-pocket per individual; $800 out-of-pocket per family (not to include deductible, mental and nervous expenses); aggregate.
APPLICATION OF COINSURANCE LIMIT: Coinsurance limit applies in the calendar year in which the limit is met and the following calendar year.
OUTPATIENT MENTAL/NERVOUS EXPENSE: 50% coinsurance while not a hospital inpatient. $500 calendar year maximum per person.
LIFETIME MAXIMUM: $1,000,000 per person.
ROOM LIMIT: Semi-private room rate.
HOSPITAL DEDUCTIBLE: Not covered.
HOME HEALTH CARE: 120 visits per calendar year. Prior hospital confinement required.
PRE-EXISTING LIMITATION: If treatment received within six months prior to effective date, $2,000 maximum payment until patient has been covered continuously under the plan for 12 months.

MEDICARE

TYPE: Coordination of Benefits.
REMARKS: Assume Medicare benefits whether or not individual enrolled. Subject to all other plan provisions.

EXCLUSIONS

1. Expenses resulting from self-inflicted injuries;
2. Work-related injuries or illnesses;
3. Services for which there is no charge in the absence of insurance;
4. Charges or services in excess of UCR or not medically necessary;
5. Charges for completion of claim forms and failure to keep appointments;
6. Routine or preventative or experimental services;
7. Eye refractions; contacts or glasses; orthotics (eye exercises); radial keratotomy or other procedures for surgical correction of refractive errors;
8. Custodial care;
9. Cosmetic surgery unless for repair of injury or surgery incurred while covered or result of mastectomy;
10. Dental care of teeth, gums, or alveolar process (TMJ) except: a) reduction of fractures of the jaw or facial bones; b) surgical correction of harelip, cleft palate, or prognathism; c) removal of salivary duct stones; d) removal of bony cysts of jaw, torus palatinus, leukoplakia, or malignant tissues;
11. Reversal of voluntary sterilization;
12. Diagnosis or treatment of infertility including artificial insemination, in vitro fertilization, etc.;
13. Contraceptive materials or devices;
14. Non-therapeutic abortions except where the life of the mother is endangered;
15. Expenses for obesity, weight reduction, or diet control unless at least 100 lbs. overweight;
16. Vitamins, food supplements, and/or protein supplements;
17. Sex-altering treatments or surgeries or related studies;
18. Orthopedic shoes or other devices for support or treatment of feet except as medically necessary following foot surgery;
19. Bio-feedback related services or treatment;
20. Experimental transplants;
21. EDTA Chelation therapy;
22. Oral Surgery.

Document 17

ROVER INSURERS, INC., 5931 ROLLING ROAD, RONSON, CO 81369, (970) 555-1369
PLAN: RED ENTERPRISES, 7677 ROYAL ROAD, COLTER, CO 81293   Effective 01/01/96
INSURANCE CONTACT: __Ravyn Ranger__   PHONE NUMBER: __(970) 555-1360__

ELIGIBILITY

EMPLOYEES must work a minimum of 30 hours per week. Eligible for coverage the first of the month following one consecutive month of continuous employment. **DEPENDENTS** eligible for coverage from birth to age 19, or to age 25 if full-time student or handicapped prior to 19/25. Is not eligible as a dependent if eligible as an employee. Unmarried natural children, legally adopted or foster children, and legal guardianship children are included. If both parents are covered by the plan, children may be covered by one parent only.

EFFECTIVE DATE

EMPLOYEE becomes effective, if written application is made prior to eligibility date, on the first of the month following 30 days of continuous employment. If employee is absent from work due to disability on the date of eligibility, coverage will not start until the first of the month following the date of return to active work. **DEPENDENTS** become effective on the date the covered employee becomes effective, if written application is made within 31 days of eligibility date. If confined in a hospital on the date of eligibility, coverage will not start until the first of the month following the date the confinement ends. Newborns are automatically covered for the first 14 days following birth. Coverage terminates after 14 days unless written application for coverage is submitted by the employee within 31 days of birth.

TERMINATION OF COVERAGE

EMPLOYEE'S coverage terminates the last day of the month following termination of employment or when the employee ceases to qualify as an eligible employee or following request for termination of coverage. **DEPENDENTS'** coverage terminates the date the employee's coverage terminates or the last day of the month during which the dependent no longer qualifies as an eligible dependent.

EXTENSION OF BENEFITS - If covered under the plan when disabled, may continue coverage in accordance with COBRA. No other extension available.

COMPREHENSIVE MEDICAL BENEFITS

PRE-ADMISSION TESTING - Outpatient diagnostic tests performed prior to inpatient admissions are paid at 100% whether through a network provider or not.

PRE-CERTIFICATION - Elective, non-emergency inpatient admissions must be approved five+ days in advance. Emergency admissions must be pre-certified within 48 hrs. of admission. Benefits are cut to 50% if not done.

SECOND SURGICAL OPINION - SSO paid at 100% of UCR. Required for the following: bunionectomy, cataract extraction, chemonucleolysis, cholecystectomy, coronary bypass, hemorrhoidectomy, hysterectomy, inguinal herniorrhaphy, laparotomy, laminectomy, mastectomy, meniscectomy, oophorectomy, prostatectomy, salpingectomy, submucous resection, total joint replacement, tenotomy, varicose veins (all procedures). **IF SSO NOT PERFORMED, ALL RELATED EXPENSES PAYABLE AT 50%**

SUPPLEMENTAL ACCIDENT EXPENSE - 100% is paid on the first $500 for services incurred within 90 days of the date of accident. Subject to $20 copayment. After $500, payments are subject to calendar year deductible. Provider does not have to be a network member to receive 100% benefit. Common accident provision applies.

OUT-PATIENT CHARGES PAYABLE AT 100% - Network out-patient facility expenses for following procedures paid 100%. Does not include professional charges: arthroscopy, breast biopsy, bronchoscopy, pilonidal cyst, myringotomy w/tubes, esophagoscopy, colonoscopy, herniorrhaphy (umbilical to age five), skin lesions (2cms+).

INDIVIDUAL CALENDAR YEAR DEDUCTIBLE	$150; three month carryover provision. All plan services subject to deductible unless otherwise indicated.
FAMILY MAX DEDUCTIBLE	$300 non-aggregate. two family members must meet individual deductible.
STANDARD COINSURANCE	80% Network; 70% Non-network.
COINSURANCE LIMIT	$1,250 out-of-pocket per individual; $2,500 out-of-pocket per family. Two individuals must meet their individual limit to satisfy family limit. Limits not to include deductible, mental/nervous expenses, or surgery expenses reduced because SSO not done. 100% of allowed amount paid thereafter for network providers; 90% for non-network providers.
LIFETIME MAXIMUM	$1,000,000 per person.
PRE-EXISTING LIMITATION	If treatment is received within 90 days prior to effective date, no coverage on that condition until continuously covered for six consecutive months from the effective date unless treatment-free for three consecutive months ending after the effective date of coverage.

INPATIENT HOSPITAL EXPENSE

DEDUCTIBLE — $200, for non-network facilities, waived for network. Inpatient hospital expenses not subject to regular Major Medical deductible.

ROOM AND BOARD — Network: 80% of semi-private/ICU; Non-network: 70% of semi-private/ICU.

MISCELLANEOUS FEES — Network: 80%; Non-network: 70%.

EXCLUSIONS — Well baby care. Automatic coverage for first seven days only if baby is ill. Otherwise, no coverage.

IF NO PRE-CERTIFICATION, ADMISSION PAID AT 50%

MENTAL/NERVOUS/PSYCHONEUROTIC

INCLUDES SUBSTANCE ABUSE AND ALCOHOLISM. Exclusions: psychological testing, hyperkinetic syndrome, learning disabilities, behavior problems, or autistic disease of childhood.

OUTPATIENT MENTAL AND NERVOUS TREATMENT

PAYABLE — $90 per visit for first five visits; $60 per visit for next 21 visits.

COINSURANCE — 80% for first five visits (maximum payable: $90/visit) 50%/visit for next 21 visits (maximum payable: $60/visit).

CALENDAR YEAR MAXIMUM — 26 visits.

INPATIENT MENTAL AND NERVOUS TREATMENT

PHYSICIAN SERVICES — 70% applies to network and non-network providers.

HOSPITAL SERVICES — 70% network and non-network providers.

DAY/PARTIAL PROGRAM — Each day in a partial/day program equals half day in an acute setting.

PROVIDERS — Psychiatrists and clinical psychologists only

MAMMOGRAMS

COINSURANCE — 80% Network; 70% Non-network.

REQUIREMENTS — Baseline mammogram for women ages 35-39; for ages 40-49, one allowed every two years; for ages 50+, one allowed every year.

X-RAY AND LABORATORY

PROFESSIONAL COMPONENTS — Professional charges paid at 25% of UCR.

DURABLE MEDICAL EQUIPMENT

COINSURANCE — 50%.

REQUIREMENTS — Prescribed by MD; must not be primarily for exercise, environmental control, convenience, comfort, or hygiene. Must be only useful for the prescribed patient. Covered up to purchase price.

MEDICARE

TYPE — Maintenance of Benefits.

REMARKS — Assume all Medicare benefits whether or not enrolled. Subject to all other plan provisions.

EXCLUSIONS

1. Expenses resulting from self-inflicted injuries;
2. Work-related injuries or illnesses;
3. Services for which there is no charge in the absence of insurance;
4. Charges or services in excess of UCR, not medically necessary, or pre-existing conditions;
5. Charges for completion of claim forms and failure to keep appointments;
6. Routine or preventative or experimental services;
7. Eye refractions; contacts or glasses; orthotics (eye exercises); radial keratotomy, or other procedures for surgical correction of refractive errors;
8. Custodial care;
9. Cosmetic surgery except repair of an injury or surgery incurred while covered or result of mastectomy;
10. Dental care of teeth, gums, or alveolar process (TMJ) except: a) reduction of fractures of the jaw or facial bones; b) surgical correction of harelip, cleft palate, prognathism; c) removal of malignant tissues;
11. Diagnosis or treatment of fertility or infertility including artificial insemination, in vitro fertilization, etc., reversal of voluntary sterilization or contraceptive materials or devices; non-therapeutic abortions;
12. Pregnancy-related expenses of dependent children for the delivery including Caesarian section. Related illnesses may be covered such as pre-eclampsia, vaginal bleeding, etc.;
13. Expenses for obesity, weight reduction, or diet control unless at least 100 lbs. overweight;
14. Vitamins, food supplements, and/or protein supplements;
15. Orthopedic shoes/devices for foot support/treatment except as medically necessary following surgery;
16. Bio-feedback related services or treatment and acupuncture treatment.

WINTER INSURANCE CO., 9763 WESTERN WAY, WHITTIER, CO 82963, (970) 555-2963
PLAN: WHITE CORPORATION, POLICY NAME: WHITE, EFFECTIVE DATE: 06/01/90
INSURANCE CONTACT: __Wilma Williams__   PHONE NUMBER: __(970) 555- 2964__

ELIGIBILITY

EMPLOYEE: Must work a minimum of 35 hours per week. Is eligible for coverage the first of the month following 60 consecutive days of continuous employment.
DEPENDENTS: Are eligible for coverage from birth to age 19, or to age 24 if a full-time student or handicapped prior to 19/24 (proof of disability must be furnished within 31 days after dependent reaches limiting age). Dependent is not eligible as a dependent if eligible as an employee. Unmarried natural children, legally adopted and foster children are included (also includes legal guardianship). If both parents are covered by the plan, children may be covered by one employee only.

EFFECTIVE DATE

EMPLOYEE: If written application is made prior to the eligibility date, coverage becomes effective the first of the month following 60 days of employment.
DEPENDENTS: The date acquired by the covered employee becomes the effective date if written application is made within 31 days of the eligibility date. Newborns are automatically covered for the first seven days following birth. Coverage will terminate after seven days unless written application for coverage is submitted by the employee within 31 days of birth.

TERMINATION OF COVERAGE

EMPLOYEE: Coverage terminates the last day of the month following termination of employment or when the employee ceases to qualify as an eligible employee, or following request for termination of coverage.
DEPENDENTS: Coverage terminates the date the employee's coverage terminates, or the last day of the month during which the dependent no longer qualifies as an eligible dependent.

EXTENSION OF BENEFITS - If covered under the plan when disabled, employee may continue coverage for 12 months following the date of termination or until no longer disabled, whichever is less.

COMPREHENSIVE MEDICAL BENEFITS

SUPPLEMENTAL ACCIDENT EXPENSE - 100% of first $300 for services incurred within 120 days of date of accident. Not subject to deductible.

PLAN BENEFITS

INDIVIDUAL CALENDAR YEAR DEDUCTIBLE: $100; three month carry-over provision.
FAMILY MAXIMUM DEDUCTIBLE: $200, aggregate.
STANDARD COINSURANCE: 90% except 100% of hospital room and board expenses for 365 days per lifetime.
COINSURANCE LIMIT: $750 out-of-pocket per individual; $1,500 out-of-pocket per family. Two separate members must satisfy the individual limit, not to include deductible, mental, or nervous expenses. Applies only in the calendar year in which the limit is met.
LIFETIME MAXIMUM: $300,000 per person.
OUTPATIENT MENTAL AND NERVOUS MAXIMUM: 30 visits per year per person (includes substance abuse and alcoholism). No inpatient maximum.
PRE-EXISTING LIMITATION: On 6/1/90 no restriction. After 6/1/90, if treatment received within 90 days prior to effective date, no coverage for that condition for 12 months from the effective date (continuously covered for 12 months) unless treatment-free for three consecutive months ending after the effective date of coverage.

X-RAY AND LABORATORY

REMARKS: Professional component charges covered at 40% of UCR allowance for procedure. Routine procedures are not covered.

INPATIENT HOSPITAL EXPENSE

Room and board payable at 100% of semi-private room rate. Miscellaneous expenses covered at 90%. Non-medically necessary, well baby care and cosmetic services excluded. Personal comfort items not covered.

MENTAL/NERVOUS/PSYCHONEUROTIC

INCLUDES SUBSTANCE ABUSE AND ALCOHOLISM. Exclusions: psychological testing.

OUTPATIENT MENTAL AND NERVOUS TREATMENT
COINSURANCE: 50% while not hospital confined.
CALENDAR YEAR MAXIMUM: None.

INPATIENT MENTAL AND NERVOUS TREATMENT
PHYSICIAN SERVICES: Covered at 90%.
HOSPITAL SERVICES: Covered at 90%.
ALLOWED PROVIDERS: Psychiatrists and clinical psychologists. Marriage and Family Child Counselor and Licensed Clinical Social Worker allowed with referral from M.D.

EXTENDED CARE FACILITY

LIFETIME MAXIMUM: 60 days.
HOSPITAL SERVICES: 80% of billed room and board charge.
REQUIREMENTS: Stay must begin within 14 days of acute hospital stay of at least three days. Extended care must be due to same disability that caused hospitalization and continued hospital care would otherwise be required.

DURABLE MEDICAL EQUIPMENT

COINSURANCE: Covered at 90%.
REQUIREMENTS: Must be prescribed by M.D. Must not be primarily necessary for exercise, environmental control, convenience, comfort or hygiene. Must only useful for the prescribed patient. Covered up to purchase price only.

REMARKS
Covered expenses include charges for the initial set of contact lenses which are necessary due to cataract surgery. Handicapped children are limited to a $15,000 lifetime maximum after attainment of age 19. Coordination of Benefits according to National Association of Insurance Carriers (NAIC) guidelines. Subject to Third Party Liability and subrogation.

MEDICARE INTEGRATION

TYPE: Non-duplication of benefits applies.
REMARKS: Assume all Medicare benefits whether or not individual actually enrolled.

EXCLUSIONS
1. Expenses resulting from self-inflicted injuries, work related injuries or illnesses;
2. Charges or services: in excess of UCR, not medically necessary, for completion of claim forms, for failure to keep appointments; for routine, preventative, or experimental services;
3. Eye refractions; contacts or glasses; orthotics (eye exercises); radial keratotomy or other procedures for surgical correction of refractive errors;
4. Custodial care and/or convalescent facility coverage;
5. Cosmetic surgery unless for repair of an injury or surgery incurred while covered or result of mastectomy;
6. Diagnosis or treatment of infertility including artificial insemination, in vitro fertilization, etc., contraceptive materials or devices, non-therapeutic abortions except where the life of the mother is endangered, reversal of voluntary sterilization;
7. Pregnancy-related expenses for dependent children;
8. Expenses for obesity, weight reduction, or diet control unless at least 100 lbs. overweight;
9. Vitamins, food supplements, and/or protein supplements;
10. Sex altering treatments or surgeries or related studies;
11. Orthopedic shoes or other devices for support or treatment of feet except as medically necessary following foot surgery;
12. Bio-feedback related services or treatment, EDTA chelation therapy.

PATIENT INFORMATION SHEET

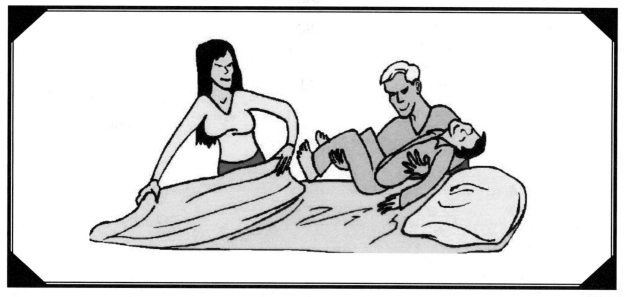

INSURED'S INFORMATION

Patient ID: _____*BEA5535-035*_____ Assigned Provider: _____ Birth date: *Feb. 10, 1965*

Name: (Last, First, Middle) *Early, Brighton* _____ Sex: ___*Male*___

Address: (Inc City, State, Zip) *1800 Liberty Lane, Colter CO 81231* _____

Home Phone: *(970) 555-3215* _____ Marital Status: *Married* _____ Social Security #: *012-12-1212* ___

Employer Name: *Blue Corporation* _____ Work Phone: *(970) 555-9876 x561* ___

Employer Address: *9817 Bobcat Blvd., Bastion, CO 81319* _____

Employment Status: ___*Full-time*___ Referred by: ____*Friend, Sherry Attricks*_____

Allergies/Medical conditions: _____

Primary Ins Name: *Ball Insurance Carriers* _____ Address: *3895 Bubble Blvd., Ste 283, Boxwood, CO 85931* ___

ID #: *021-12-1212* _____ Plan #/Name: *98135 Blue* _____ Policy Holder Name: *Brighton Early* ___

Secondary Ins Name: ___*See Wife*___ Address: _____

ID #: _____ Plan #/Name: _____ Policy Holder Name: _____

SPOUSE'S INFORMATION

Patient ID: ___*NEA5536-036*_____ Assigned Provider: _____ Birth date: *Apr. 1, 1968*

Name: (Last, First, Middle) *Early, Neva Tu* _____ Sex: ___*Female*___

Social Security #: *112-12-1122* _____ Employment Status: ___*Full-time*_____

Employer Name: *White Corporation* _____ Work Phone: *(970) 555-1234* ___

Employer Address: ____*1234 Whitaker Lane, Colter, CO 81250*_____

Allergies/Medical conditions: ___*Insurance effective 3/1/97*_____

Primary Ins Name: *Winter Insurance Co.* _____ Address: *9763 Western Way, Whittier, CO 82963* ___

ID #: *112-12-Whi* _____ Plan #/Name: *White Corp.* _____ Policy Holder Name: *Neva Tu Early* ___

Secondary Ins Name: ___*See Husband*___ Address: _____

ID #: _____ Plan #/Name: _____ Policy Holder Name: _____

CHILD #1

Patient ID: _BTI5537-037_   Assigned Provider: _____   Birth date: _Jul. 1, 1989_

Name of Minor Child: _Tired, Barry_   Social Security #: _102-12-0701_

Sex: _Male_   Marital Status: _Single_   Relationship to Insured: _step-son (Larry)/ son_

Allergies/Medical conditions: _____

Primary Ins Name: _Step-Father/Mother/Father?_   Address: _See below_

Secondary Ins Name: _Step-Father/Mother/Father?_   Address: _See below_

CHILD #2

Patient ID: _IEA5538-038_   Assigned Provider: _____   Birth date: _Nov. 4, 1994_

Name of Minor Child: _Early, Ivanna B._   Social Security #: _112-02-1104_

Sex: _Female_   Marital Status: _Single_   Relationship to Insured: _Child (of both)_

Allergies/Medical conditions: _____

Primary Ins Name: _Father/ Mother?_   Address: _____

Secondary Ins Name: _Father/ Mother?_   Address: _____

CHILD #3

Patient ID: _____   Assigned Provider: _____   Birth date: _____

Name of Minor Child: _____   Social Security #: _____

Sex: _____   Marital Status: _____   Relationship to Insured: _____

Allergies/Medical conditions: _____

Primary Ins Name: _____   Primary Insured: _____

Secondary Ins Name: _____   Secondary Insured: _____

EMERGENCY CONTACT

Name: _Ian Tired_   Home Phone: _(970) 555-7007_   Other Phone _(970) 555-9009_

Address: (Inc City, State, Zip)   _3758 Mattress Drive, Mayhem, CO 81245_

ACKNOWLEDGMENT AND AUTHORITY FOR TREATMENT AND PAYMENT

_BE_   I consent to treatment as necessary or desirable to the care of the patient named above, including but not restricted to whatever drugs, medicine, performance of operations and conduct of laboratory, x-ray, or other studies that may be used by the attending doctor, his/her nurse or qualified designate:

_BE_   I also acknowledge full responsibility for the payment of such services and agree to pay for them upon demand, in full, AT THE TIME OF SERVICE. If the physician must use a collection agency/attorney or court to collect its charges, then I will pay reasonable attorney fees and costs incurred in collecting same, regardless of insurance coverage.

_BE_   I hereby authorize payment directly to Consolidated Health Services of the medical expense benefits otherwise payable to me but not to exceed my indebtedness to said physician on account of the enclosed charge.

_BE_   I hereby authorize any medical practitioner, medical or medically related facility, insurance or reinsuring company, consumer reporting agency, or employer having information with respect to any physical or mental condition and/or treatment of me or my minor children and any other non-medical information of me and my minor children to give to the group policy holder, my employer, or its legal representative, any and all such information.

_BE_   I understand the information obtained by the use of the Authorization will be used to determine eligibility for insurance, and eligibility for benefits under any existing policy. Any information obtained will not be released by/to any organization EXCEPT to the group policyholder, my employer, reinsuring companies, the Medical Information Bureau, Inc., or other persons or organizations performing business or legal services in connection with my application, claim, or as may be otherwise lawfully required or as I may further authorize.

_BE_   I further agree that a photographic copy of this Authorization shall be valid as the original. This Authorization shall be valid for one year from the date shown below.

Signature of Insured: _Brighton Early_   Date: _Jan. 21, 20XX_

Signature of Spouse: _____   Date: _____

I'm not sure whose insurance would pay first or second for the kids. Barry also has insurance through his father (Neva's first husband), and his new wife. Their information is: Father: Ian Tired, 39458 Mattress Drive, Mayhem, CO 81245. SSN: 121-00-1212, born January 30, 1965. Employer: Blue Corp (Ball Insurance Carriers) policy #121-00-1212, Group # 98135 Blue. Stepmother: Bea Tired, SSN: 000-12-0012, born January 30, 1964. Employer: Purple Players Inc., 3165 Peanut Place, Passion, CO 82369 (970) 555-9632. Insurance Carrier: Peacock Insurers, 5613 Proud Plaza, Princeton, CO 83659 (970) 555-3683.

PATIENT INFORMATION SHEET

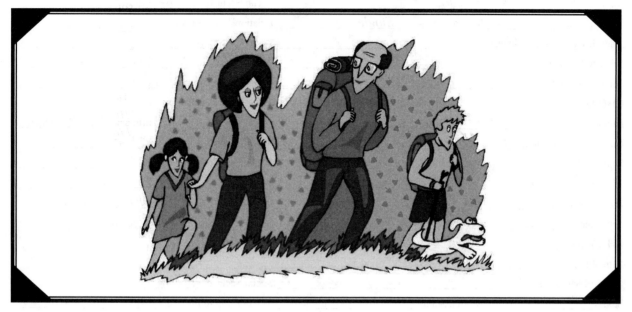

INSURED'S INFORMATION

Patient ID: _CFE5539-039_ Assigned Provider: _____ Birth date: _Aug. 17, 1952_

Name: (Last, First, Middle) _Fever, Cab N._ Sex: _Male_

Address: (Inc City, State, Zip) _1432 Nightmare Way, Apt #99, Colter, CO 81352_

Home Phone: _(970) 555-1432_ Marital Status: _Married_ Social Security #: _014-99-1414_

Employer Name: _Red Enterprises_ Work Phone: _____

Employer Address: _7677 Royal Road, Colter, CO 81293_

Employment Status: _Full-time_ Referred by: _PPO List_

Allergies/Medical conditions: _____

Primary Ins Name: _Rover Insurers Inc._ Address: _5931 Rolling Road, Ronson, CO 81369_

ID #: _014-99-Red_ Plan #/Name: _41935 Red_ Policy Holder Name: _Cab N. Fever_

Secondary Ins Name: _See Wife_ Address: _____

ID #: _____ Plan #/Name: _____ Policy Holder Name: _____

SPOUSE'S INFORMATION

Patient ID: _EFE5540-040_ Assigned Provider: _____ Birth date: _Aug. 12, 1964_

Name: (Last, First, Middle) _Fever, Elle O._ Sex: _Female_

Social Security #: _014-67-1764_ Employment Status: _Full-time_

Employer Name: _Blue Corporation_ Work Phone: _(970) 555-9876_

Employer Address: _9817 Bobcat Blvd., Bastion, CO 81319_

Allergies/Medical conditions: _____

Primary Ins Name: _Ball Insurance Carriers_ Address: _3895 Bubble Blvd. Ste. 283, Boxwood, CO 85931_

ID #: _014-67-1764_ Plan #/Name: _98135Blue_ Policy Holder Name: _Elle O. Fever_

Secondary Ins Name: _See Husband_ Address: _____

ID #: _____ Plan #/Name: _____ Policy Holder Name: _____

CHILD #1

Patient ID: ___SFE5541-041___ Assigned Provider: _____ Birth date: _Dec. 19, 1994_

Name of Minor Child: _Fever, Scarlet_____ Social Security #: _114-19-6385_____

Sex: _Female_____ Marital Status: ___Single_____ Relationship to Insured: _Daughter_____

Allergies/Medical conditions: _____

Primary Ins Name: _____ Primary Insured: ____Father or Mother?____

Secondary Ins Name: _____ Secondary Insured: ___Father or Mother?___

CHILD #2

Patient ID: ___TFE5542-042___ Assigned Provider: _____ Birth date: _Nov. 23, 1996_

Name of Minor Child: _Fever, Ty Phoid_____ Social Security #: _114-23-1740_____

Sex: _Male_____ Marital Status: ___Single_____ Relationship to Insured: _Son_____

Allergies/Medical conditions: _____

Primary Ins Name: _____ Primary Insured: ____Father or Mother?____

Secondary Ins Name: _____ Secondary Insured: ___Father or Mother?___

CHILD #3

Patient ID: _____ Assigned Provider: _____ Birth date: _____

Name of Minor Child: _____ Social Security #: _____

Sex: _____ Marital Status: _____ Relationship to Insured: _____

Allergies/Medical conditions: _____

Primary Ins Name: _____ Primary Insured: _____

Secondary Ins Name: _____ Secondary Insured: _____

EMERGENCY CONTACT

Name: _Hy Fever_____ Home Phone: _(970) 555-3353___ Other Phone: _(970) 555-1100___

Address: (Inc City, State, Zip)____1432 Nightmare Way, Apt #95, Colter, CO 81352_____

ACKNOWLEDGMENT AND AUTHORITY FOR TREATMENT AND PAYMENT

___CF___ I consent to treatment as necessary or desirable to the care of the patient named above, including but not restricted to whatever drugs, medicine, performance of operations and conduct of laboratory, x-ray, or other studies that may be used by the attending doctor, his/her nurse or qualified designate:

___CF___ I also acknowledge full responsibility for the payment of such services and agree to pay for them upon demand, in full, AT THE TIME OF SERVICE. If the physician must use a collection agency/attorney or court to collect its charges, then I will pay reasonable attorney fees and costs incurred in collecting same, regardless of insurance coverage.

___CF___ I hereby authorize payment directly to Consolidated Health Services of the medical expense benefits otherwise payable to me but not to exceed my indebtedness to said physician on account of the enclosed charge.

___CF___ I hereby authorize any medical practitioner, medical or medically related facility, insurance or reinsuring company, consumer reporting agency, or employer having information with respect to any physical or mental condition and/or treatment of me or my minor children and any other non-medical information of me and my minor children to give to the group policy holder, my employer, or its legal representative, any and all such information.

___CF___ I understand the information obtained by the use of the Authorization will be used to determine eligibility for insurance, and eligibility for benefits under any existing policy. Any information obtained will not be released by/to any organization EXCEPT to the group policyholder, my employer, reinsuring companies, the Medical Information Bureau, Inc., or other persons or organizations performing business or legal services in connection with my application, claim, or as may be otherwise lawfully required or as I may further authorize.

___CF___ I further agree that a photographic copy of this Authorization shall be valid as the original. This Authorization shall be valid for one year from the date shown below.

Signature of Insured: ___Cab N. Fever_____ Date: ___Jan. 21, 20XX_____

Signature of Spouse: _____ Date: _____

Document 21

OFFICE VISIT PROCEDURES

DESCRIPTION	TIME	CHARGE
NEW PATIENT OFFICE VISITS		
Problem focused history/exam, straightforward	20 min	$85
Expanded history/exam, straightforward	30 min	$95
Detailed history/exam, low complexity	40 min	$105
Comprehensive history/exam, moderate complexity	45 min	$120
Comprehensive history/exam, high complexity	60 min	$135
ESTABLISHED PATIENT OFFICE VISITS		
Minimal visit	10 min	$50
Problem focused history/exam, straightforward	15 min	$55
Expanded history/exam, low complexity	20 min	$80
Detailed history/exam, moderate complexity	25 min	$95
Comprehensive history/exam, high complexity	30 min	$105

PATIENT INFORMATION SHEET

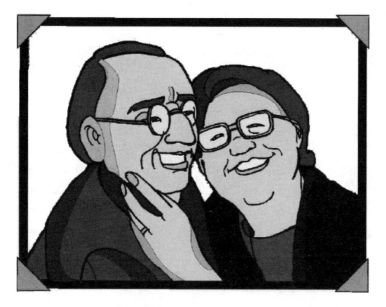

INSURED'S INFORMATION

Patient ID: __SHA5543-043__   Assigned Provider: _____   Birth date: _Jan. 15, 1920_

Name: (Last, First, Middle) __Hart, Shay Kee_____   Sex: ___Male_____

Address: (Inc City, State, Zip) _2093 Garden Way, Colter, CO 81223_____

Home Phone: _(970) 555-9600_____   Marital Status: _Married_____   Social Security #: _713-77-7700_____

Employer Name: __Red Enterprises_____   Work Phone: _(970) 555-0863_____

Employer Address: _7677 Royal Road, Colter, CO 81293_____

Employment Status: ___Retired_____   Referred by: ___PPO List_____

Allergies/Medical conditions: ___Lou Gehrig's Disease_____

Primary Ins Name: _Medicare_____   Address: _1873 Montrose Ave., Minx, CO 82377_____

ID #: _713-77-7700A____   Plan #/Name: _____   Policy Holder Name: _Shay Kee Hart_____

Secondary Ins Name: __Rover Insurers, Inc._____   Address: _5931 Rolling Road, Ronson, CO 81369___

ID #:_____   Plan #/Name: _41935Red-Medigap_ Policy Holder Name: _Shay Kee Hart_____

SPOUSE'S INFORMATION

Patient ID: __BHA5545-045____   Assigned Provider: _____   Birth date: _Dec. 18, 1922_

Name: (Last, First, Middle) __Hart, Brooke N._____   Sex: ___Female____

Social Security #: __717-71-7171_____   Employment Status: __Retired Homemaker_____

Employer Name: _____   Work Phone:_____

Employer Address: _____

Allergies/Medical conditions: _____

Primary Ins Name: _Medicare_____   Address: _1873 Montrose Ave., Minx, CO 82377_____

ID #: _713-77-7700A____   Plan #/Name: _____   Policy Holder Name: _Shay Kee Hart_____

Secondary Ins Name: __Rover Insurers, Inc._____   Address: _5931 Rolling Road, Ronson, CO 81369___

ID #: _____   Plan #/Name: _41935Red-Medigap_ Policy Holder Name: _Shay Kee Hart_____

CHILD #1

Patient ID: _____ Assigned Provider: _____ Birth date: _____

Name of Minor Child: _____ Social Security #: _____

Sex: _____ Marital Status: _____ Relationship to Insured: _____

Allergies/Medical conditions: _____

Primary Ins Name: _____ Primary Insured: _____

Secondary Ins Name: _____ Secondary Insured: _____

CHILD #2

Patient ID: _____ Assigned Provider: _____ Birth date: _____

Name of Minor Child: _____ Social Security #: _____

Sex: _____ Marital Status: _____ Relationship to Insured: _____

Allergies/Medical conditions: _____

Primary Ins Name: _____ Primary Insured: _____

Secondary Ins Name: _____ Secondary Insured: _____

CHILD #3

Patient ID: _____ Assigned Provider: _____ Birth date: _____

Name of Minor Child: _____ Social Security #: _____

Sex: _____ Marital Status: _____ Relationship to Insured: _____

Allergies/Medical conditions: _____

Primary Ins Name: _____ Primary Insured: _____

Secondary Ins Name: _____ Secondary Insured: _____

EMERGENCY CONTACT

Name: *E. K. Gee*_____ Home Phone: *(970) 555- 6452*_____ Other Phone: *(970) 555- 3008*_____

Address: (Inc City, State, Zip)____*752 Forest Drive Colter, CO 81223*_____

ACKNOWLEDGMENT AND AUTHORITY FOR TREATMENT AND PAYMENT

SKH   I consent to treatment as necessary or desirable to the care of the patient named above, including but not restricted to whatever drugs, medicine, performance of operations and conduct of laboratory, x-ray, or other studies that may be used by the attending doctor, his/her nurse or qualified designate:

SKH   I also acknowledge full responsibility for the payment of such services and agree to pay for them upon demand, in full, AT THE TIME OF SERVICE. If the physician must use a collection agency/attorney or court to collect its charges, then I will pay reasonable attorney fees and costs incurred in collecting same, regardless of insurance coverage.

SKH   I hereby authorize payment directly to Consolidated Health Services of the medical expense benefits otherwise payable to me but not to exceed my indebtedness to said physician on account of the enclosed charge.

SKH   I hereby authorize any medical practitioner, medical or medically related facility, insurance or reinsuring company, consumer reporting agency, or employer having information with respect to any physical or mental condition and/or treatment of me or my minor children and any other non-medical information of me and my minor children to give to the group policy holder, my employer, or its legal representative, any and all such information.

SKH   I understand the information obtained by the use of the Authorization will be used to determine eligibility for insurance, and eligibility for benefits under any existing policy. Any information obtained will not be released by/to any organization EXCEPT to the group policyholder, my employer, reinsuring companies, the Medical Information Bureau, Inc., or other persons or organizations performing business or legal services in connection with my application, claim, or as may be otherwise lawfully required or as I may further authorize.

SKH   I further agree that a photographic copy of this Authorization shall be valid as the original. This Authorization shall be valid for one year from the date shown below.

Signature of Insured: ___*Shay Kee Hart*_____ Date: ___*Jan. 21, 20XX*_____

Signature of Spouse: _____ Date: _____

TYPE	PROCDR CODE	DESCRIPTION
A	HRDSHP	Write-off due to patient's financial hardship.
A	DEC	Amount written off due to death of patient.
A	CHG ERR	Amount changed due to an error in the original charge. This can be a negative or a positive adjustment (i.e., a lessor or higher amount added to the original charge).
A	CODE ERR	Amount changed or deleted due to an error in the procedure code entry. This adjustment would be best served by adjusting out the old charge and entering the new procedure code.
A	PT REQ	Amount adjusted due to patient demand. (This code may be used to adjust a cost if the patient is dissatisfied with service and/or insists the charge is excessive for the services rendered.)
A	CTSY FAM	Amount adjusted as a patient courtesy due to patient's familial relationship to another Consolidated Health Services provider.
A	DISC PT	Patient has discontinued treatment with this provider and there is no hope of recovering payment.
A	PT UNK	Patient address, phone, and other information are unknown (i.e., patient has moved and left no forwarding address). Efforts to trace patient have been unsuccessful.
B	INS DWNCD	Insurance downcoded charges. The insurance carrier ruled that the procedures rendered did not justify the higher code level.
B	MCR APP	Amount adjusted to conform to Medicare's approved amount.

NOTE: All providers should break down adjustments to prevent a loss of time. In an audit situation, the auditors will need to know the reason behind each of the adjustments.

PATIENT INFORMATION SHEET

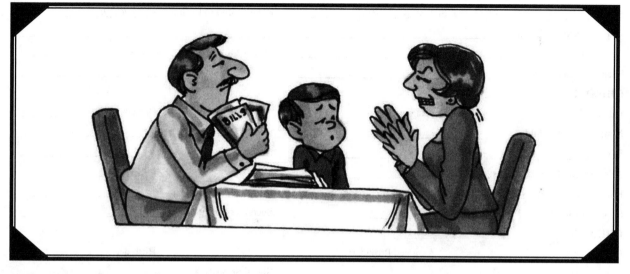

INSURED'S INFORMATION

Patient ID: _BFI5546-046_   Assigned Provider: _____ Birth date: _Nov. 24, 1969_

Name: (Last, First, Middle) _Fraide, B.A._   Sex: _Male_

Address: (Inc City, State, Zip) _9009 Marble Manor Lane, Colton, CO 81956_

Home Phone: _(970) 555-1959_   Marital Status: _Married_   Social Security #: _013-13-1313_

Employer Name: _Rocky Corporation_   Work Phone: _(970) 555-0846_

Employer Address: _1234 Ribbon Road, Rudolph, CO 81208_

Employment Status: _Full-time_   Referred by: _Yellow Pages Ad_

Allergies/Medical conditions: _____

Primary Ins Name: _Summer Insurance Co._   Address: _18932 Spring Road, Autumn, CO 82974_

ID #: _111-11-HMO_   Plan #/Name: _Rocky Company_   Policy Holder Name: _B. A. Fraide_

Secondary Ins Name: _N/A_   Address: _____

ID #: _____ Plan #/Name: _____ Policy Holder Name: _____

SPOUSE'S INFORMATION

Patient ID: _NFI5547-047_   Assigned Provider: _____ Birth date: _Jun. 13, 1966_

Name: (Last, First, Middle) _Fraide, Nada_   Sex: _Female_

Social Security #: _013-56-0613_   Employment Status: _Part-time_

Employer Name: _Red Enterprises_   Work Phone: _(970) 555-0863_

Employer Address: _7677 Royal Road, Colter, CO 81293_

Allergies/Medical conditions: _____

Primary Ins Name: _See Husband_   Address: _____

ID #: _____ Plan #/Name: _____ Policy Holder Name: _____

Secondary Ins Name: _N/A_   Address: _____

ID #: _____ Plan #/Name: _____ Policy Holder Name: _____

CHILD #1

Patient ID: _JFI5548-048_   Assigned Provider: _____   Birth date: _May. 7, 1997_

Name of Minor Child: _Fraide, Jose_   Social Security #: _013-22-2013_

Sex: _Male_   Marital Status: _Single_   Relationship to Insured: _Son (adopted)_

Allergies/Medical conditions: _____

Primary Ins Name: _____   Primary Insured: _Father_

Secondary Ins Name: _____   Secondary Insured: _____

CHILD #2

Patient ID: _____   Assigned Provider: _____   Birth date: _____

Name of Minor Child: _____   Social Security #: _____

Sex: _____   Marital Status: _____   Relationship to Insured: _____

Allergies/Medical conditions: _____

Primary Ins Name: _____   Primary Insured: _____

Secondary Ins Name: _____   Secondary Insured: _____

CHILD #3

Patient ID: _____   Assigned Provider: _____   Birth date: _____

Name of Minor Child: _____   Social Security #: _____

Sex: _____   Marital Status: _____   Relationship to Insured: _____

Allergies/Medical conditions: _____

Primary Ins Name: _____   Primary Insured: _____

Secondary Ins Name: _____   Secondary Insured: _____

EMERGENCY CONTACT

Name: _Virginia Wolfe_   Home Phone: _(970) 555-1298_   Other Phone: _(970) 555-5499_

Address: (Inc City, State, Zip) _9515 Filthy Lane, Colton, CO 81956_

ACKNOWLEDGMENT AND AUTHORITY FOR TREATMENT AND PAYMENT

_BF_   I consent to treatment as necessary or desirable to the care of the patient named above, including but not restricted to whatever drugs, medicine, performance of operations and conduct of laboratory, x-ray, or other studies that may be used by the attending doctor, his/her nurse or qualified designate:

_BF_   I also acknowledge full responsibility for the payment of such services and agree to pay for them upon demand, in full, AT THE TIME OF SERVICE. If the physician must use a collection agency/attorney or court to collect its charges, then I will pay reasonable attorney fees and costs incurred in collecting same, regardless of insurance coverage.

_BF_   I hereby authorize payment directly to Consolidated Health Services of the medical expense benefits otherwise payable to me but not to exceed my indebtedness to said physician on account of the enclosed charge.

_BF_   I hereby authorize any medical practitioner, medical or medically related facility, insurance or reinsuring company, consumer reporting agency, or employer having information with respect to any physical or mental condition and/or treatment of me or my minor children and any other non-medical information of me and my minor children to give to the group policy holder, my employer, or its legal representative, any and all such information.

_BF_   I understand the information obtained by the use of the Authorization will be used to determine eligibility for insurance, and eligibility for benefits under any existing policy. Any information obtained will not be released by/to any organization EXCEPT to the group policyholder, my employer, reinsuring companies, the Medical Information Bureau, Inc., or other persons or organizations performing business or legal services in connection with my application, claim, or as may be otherwise lawfully required or as I may further authorize.

_BF_   I further agree that a photographic copy of this Authorization shall be valid as the original. This Authorization shall be valid for one year from the date shown below.

Signature of Insured: _B.A. Fraide_   Date: _Jan. 21, 20XX_

Signature of Spouse: _Nada Fraide_   Date: _Jan. 21, 20XX_

WINTER INSURANCE
9763 WESTERN WAY
WHITTIER, CO 82963

PATIENT NAME	DATE OF SERVICE	PROCEDURE	BILLED AMOUNT	ALLOWED AMOUNT	% OF AMOUNT	PAYMENT AMOUNT	DENIED AMOUNT	REASON CODE
POOLE, CARLA	01/08/XX	ER VISIT	$ 55.00	$ 50.00	100%*	$ 50.00	$ 5.00	45
O'GEN, OX	01/14/XX	OFFICE VISIT	$ 55.00	$ 50.00	90%	$ 0.00**	$ 5.00	45
POOLE, GENE	01/08/XX	HOSP CONSULT	$310.00	$274.00	90%	$156.60**	$ 36.00	45
	01/09-10/XX	HOSPITAL VISIT	$150.00	$100.00	90%	$ 90.00	$ 50.00	45
	01/11/XX	HOSPITAL D/C	$150.00	$118.00	90%	$106.20	$ 32.00	45
TOTAL			$610.00	$492.00		$352.80	$118.00	
DUNNITT, D. JOBB	01/09/XX	PENDED						
TOTALS			$720.00	$592.00		$402.80	$128.00	

REASON CODES:

45   BILLED AMOUNT EXCEEDS AMOUNT ALLOWED BY THE PLAN.

*   ACCIDENT BENEFIT AMOUNT

**   APPLIED TOWARD DEDUCTIBLE

DETACH CHECK BEFORE CASHING

WINTER INSURANCE
9763 WESTERN WAY
WHITTIER, CO 82963

BANK OF COLORS
Whittier Branch
2300 Whyme Way
Whittier, CO 82963

(970) 555-5555

1111
33-77
1293

January 24,   20 XX

DOLLARS $ 402.80

PAY   Four Hundred Two and 80/100

TO
THE
ORDER
OF
Consolidated Health Services
1357 Castle Blvd, Suite 515
Colter, CO 81222-2222

William Windsor

⑈001111⑈ ⑆111000123⑆ 0123 4567⑈ ⑈0000011123⑈

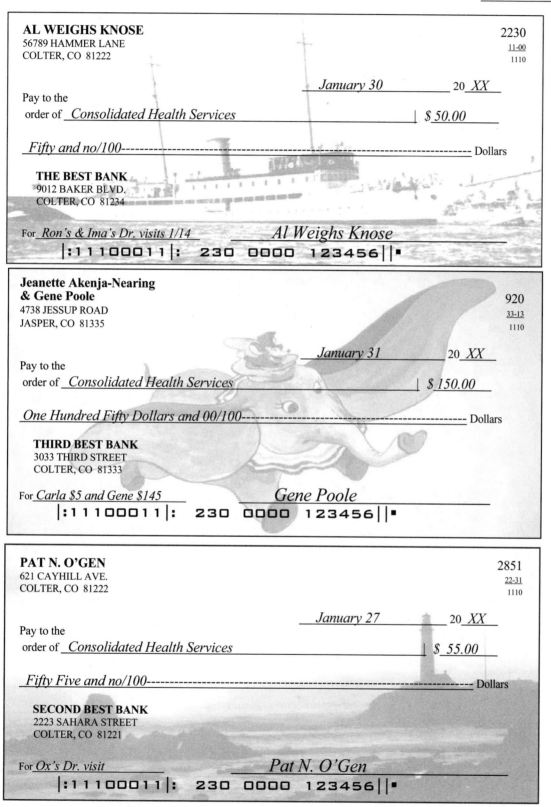

AL WEIGHS KNOSE
56789 HAMMER LANE
COLTER, CO 81222

2230

11-00
1110

January 30   20 *XX*

Pay to the
order of *Consolidated Health Services* $ *50.00*

Fifty and no/100-- Dollars

THE BEST BANK
9012 BAKER BLVD.
COLTER, CO 81234

For *Ron's & Ima's Dr. visits 1/14*   *Al Weighs Knose*

|:11100011|:   230   0000   123456||▪

**Jeanette Akenja-Nearing
& Gene Poole**
4738 JESSUP ROAD
JASPER, CO 81335

920

33-13
1110

January 31   20 *XX*

Pay to the
order of *Consolidated Health Services* $ *150.00*

One Hundred Fifty Dollars and 00/100--- Dollars

THIRD BEST BANK
3033 THIRD STREET
COLTER, CO 81333

For *Carla $5 and Gene $145*   *Gene Poole*

|:11100011|:   230   0000   123456||▪

PAT N. O'GEN
621 CAYHILL AVE.
COLTER, CO 81222

2851

22-31
1110

January 27   20 *XX*

Pay to the
order of *Consolidated Health Services* $ *55.00*

Fifty Five and no/100-- Dollars

SECOND BEST BANK
2223 SAHARA STREET
COLTER, CO 81221

For *Ox's Dr. visit*   *Pat N. O'Gen*

|:11100011|:   230   0000   123456||▪

ROVER INSURERS INC.
5931 ROLLING ROAD
RONSON, CO 81369

PATIENT NAME	DATE OF SERVICE	PROCEDURE	BILLED AMOUNT	ALLOWED AMOUNT	% OF AMOUNT	PAYMENT AMOUNT	DENIED AMOUNT	REASON CODE
THEROAD, KENT C.	01/09/XX	OPTHAL VISIT	$100.00	$75.00	80%	$0.00*	$25.00	36
	01/09/XX	BLOOD SPECIMEN	$15.00	$7.50	80%	$0.00*	$7.50	36
	TOTAL		$115.00	$82.50		$0.00	$32.50	
PENDENT, DEE	01/14/XX	OFFICE VISIT	$35.00	$35.00	80%	$8.00**	$0.00	
ALLITY, MORT	01/04/XX	HOSP ADMIT	$110.00	$85.00	80%	$0.00*	$25.00	36
	01/05-07/XX	HOSP VISITS	$285.00	$225.00	80%	$128.00	$60.00	36
	01/08/XX	HOSP D/C	$115.00	$80.00	80%	$64.00	$35.00	36
	TOTAL		$510.00	$390.00		$192.00	$120.00	
PENDENT, DEE	01/03/XX	HOSP ADMIT	$250.00	$187.00	80%	$149.60	$63.00	36
	01/07-08/XX	HOSP VISITS	$165.00	$144.00	80%	$115.20	$21.00	36
	01/09/XX	HOSP D/C	$115.00	$115.00	80%	$92.00	$0.00	36
	TOTAL		$530.00	$446.00		$356.80	$84.00	
TOTALS			$1,190.00	$953.50		$556.80	$236.50	

REASON CODES:

36   BILLED AMOUNT EXCEEDS AMOUNT ALLOWED BY THE PLAN.

** $25 LEFT ON DEDUCTIBLE AFTER CARRY-OVER DEDUCTIBLE CALCULATED

*   APPLIED TOWARD DEDUCTIBLE

DETACH CHECK BEFORE CASHING

ROVER INSURERS, INC.
5931 ROLLING ROAD
RONSON, CO 81369

04-9999

$\underline{08-12}$
1100

BANK OF COLORS   (970) 555-5555
Ronson Branch
2300 Rocky Road
Ronson, CO 81369

January 31,   20 XX

PAY   Five Hundred Fifty Six and 80/100   DOLLARS $ 556.80

TO THE ORDER OF

Consolidated Health Services
1357 Castle Blvd, Suite 515
Colter, CO 81222-2222

Randy Rover

⑈001111⑈ ⑈:111000123⑈: 0123 4567⑈⑈

⑈0000011123⑈⑈

BALL INSURANCE CARRIERS
3895 BUBBLE BLVD.
BOXWOOD, CO 85926

PATIENT NAME	DATE OF SERVICE	PROCEDURE	BILLED AMOUNT	ALLOWED AMOUNT	BASIC AMOUNT	PAYMENT AMOUNT	DENIED AMOUNT	REASON CODE
ATTRICKS, PETEY	01/14/XX	OFFICE VISIT	$190.00	$148.00	8.50	$ 11.60**	$ 42.00	19
	01/14/XX	BLOOD SAMPLE	$ 15.00	$ 7.50	.20	$ 5.84	$ 7.50	19
	TOTAL		$205.00	$155.50	8.70	$ 17.44	$ 49.50	
ATTRICKS, PETEY	01/14/XX	COMP CONSULT	$275.00	$225.00	12.75	$169.80	$ 50.00	19
	TOTAL		$275.00	$225.00	12.75	$169.80	$ 50.00	
TOTALS			$480.00	$380.50	21.45	$187.24	$ 99.50	

REASON CODES:

19   BILLED AMOUNT EXCEEDS AMOUNT ALLOWED BY THE PLAN.

*   ACCIDENT BENEFIT AMOUNT

**   APPLIED TOWARD DEDUCTIBLE

DETACH CHECK BEFORE CASHING

BALL INSURANCE CARRIERS
3895 BUBBLE BLVD.
BOXWOOD, CO 85926

BANK OF COLORS (970) 555-5555
Boxwood Branch
2300 Barker Blvd.
Boxwood, CO 85926

12341
01-11
1000

January 31,   20 XX

PAY   Two Hundred Eight and 69/100   DOLLARS $ 208.69

TO THE ORDER OF   Consolidated Health Services
1357 Castle Blvd, Suite 515
Colter, CO 81222-2222

Bob Brader

⑆001111⑆ ⑆111000123⑆ 0123   4567⑆   ⑆000011123⑆

Document 29

Codie Pendent
1501 Darning Drive
Durham, CO 81235

January 31, 20XX

Dr. Phil Goode
1357 Castle Blvd., Ste 501
Colter, CO 81222

Dear Dr. Goode:

My daughter Dee and I recently moved. Please note the following change of address for your records:

Moved from: 1111 E. Dunphy Ave.
                     Colter, CO 81222

Moved to: 1501 Darning Drive
                     Durham, CO 81235

Please forward all bills and information concerning our account to this new address.

Thank you very much.

Sincerely,

Codie Pendent
Codie Pendent

Document 30

PATIENT INFORMATION SHEET

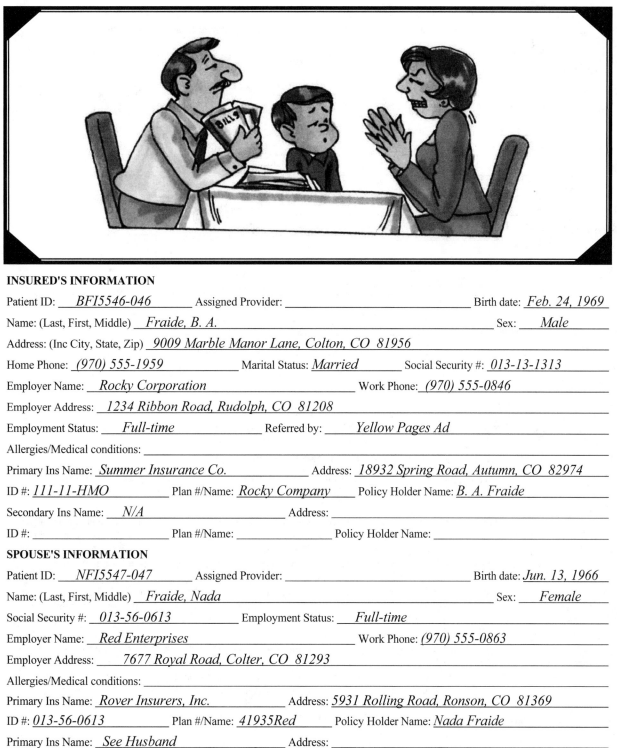

INSURED'S INFORMATION

Patient ID: *BFI5546-046*   Assigned Provider: _____   Birth date: *Feb. 24, 1969*

Name: (Last, First, Middle) *Fraide, B. A.*   Sex: *Male*

Address: (Inc City, State, Zip) *9009 Marble Manor Lane, Colton, CO 81956*

Home Phone: *(970) 555-1959*   Marital Status: *Married*   Social Security #: *013-13-1313*

Employer Name: *Rocky Corporation*   Work Phone: *(970) 555-0846*

Employer Address: *1234 Ribbon Road, Rudolph, CO 81208*

Employment Status: *Full-time*   Referred by: *Yellow Pages Ad*

Allergies/Medical conditions: _____

Primary Ins Name: *Summer Insurance Co.*   Address: *18932 Spring Road, Autumn, CO 82974*

ID #: *111-11-HMO*   Plan #/Name: *Rocky Company*   Policy Holder Name: *B. A. Fraide*

Secondary Ins Name: *N/A*   Address: _____

ID #: _____   Plan #/Name: _____   Policy Holder Name: _____

SPOUSE'S INFORMATION

Patient ID: *NFI5547-047*   Assigned Provider: _____   Birth date: *Jun. 13, 1966*

Name: (Last, First, Middle) *Fraide, Nada*   Sex: *Female*

Social Security #: *013-56-0613*   Employment Status: *Full-time*

Employer Name: *Red Enterprises*   Work Phone: *(970) 555-0863*

Employer Address: *7677 Royal Road, Colter, CO 81293*

Allergies/Medical conditions: _____

Primary Ins Name: *Rover Insurers, Inc.*   Address: *5931 Rolling Road, Ronson, CO 81369*

ID #: *013-56-0613*   Plan #/Name: *41935Red*   Policy Holder Name: *Nada Fraide*

Primary Ins Name: *See Husband*   Address: _____

ID #: _____   Plan #/Name: _____   Policy Holder Name: _____

CHILD #1

Patient ID: _JF15548-048_   Assigned Provider: _____   Birth date: _May. 7, 1997_

Name of Minor Child: _Fraide, Jose_   Social Security #: _013-22-2013_

Sex: _Male_   Marital Status: _Single_   Relationship to Insured: _Son (adopted)_

Allergies/Medical conditions: _____

Primary Ins Name: _____   Primary Insured: _Father or Mother?_

Secondary Ins Name: _____   Secondary Insured: _Father or Mother?_

CHILD #2   _How do we know whose insurance is primary or secondary? Please fix this for us._

Patient ID: _____   Assigned Provider: _____   Birth date: _____

Name of Minor Child: _____   Social Security #: _____

Sex: _____   Marital Status: _____   Relationship to Insured: _____

Allergies/Medical conditions: _____

Primary Ins Name: _____   Primary Insured: _____

Secondary Ins Name: _____   Secondary Insured: _____

CHILD #3

Patient ID: _____   Assigned Provider: _____   Birth date: _____

Name of Minor Child: _____   Social Security #: _____

Sex: _____   Marital Status: _____   Relationship to Insured: _____

Allergies/Medical conditions: _____

Primary Ins Name: _____   Primary Insured: _____

Secondary Ins Name: _____   Secondary Insured: _____

EMERGENCY CONTACT

Name: _Virginia Wolfe_   Home Phone: _(970) 555-1298_   Other Phone: _(970) 555-5499_

Address: (Inc City, State, Zip) _9515 Filthy Lane, Colton, CO 81956_

ACKNOWLEDGMENT AND AUTHORITY FOR TREATMENT AND PAYMENT

_BF_   I consent to treatment as necessary or desirable to the care of the patient named above, including but not restricted to whatever drugs, medicine, performance of operations and conduct of laboratory, x-ray, or other studies that may be used by the attending doctor, his/her nurse or qualified designate:

_BF_   I also acknowledge full responsibility for the payment of such services and agree to pay for them upon demand, in full, AT THE TIME OF SERVICE. If the physician must use a collection agency/attorney or court to collect its charges, then I will pay reasonable attorney fees and costs incurred in collecting same, regardless of insurance coverage.

_BF_   I hereby authorize payment directly to Consolidated Health Services of the medical expense benefits otherwise payable to me but not to exceed my indebtedness to said physician on account of the enclosed charge.

_BF_   I hereby authorize any medical practitioner, medical or medically related facility, insurance or reinsuring company, consumer reporting agency, or employer having information with respect to any physical or mental condition and/or treatment of me or my minor children and any other non-medical information of me and my minor children to give to the group policy holder, my employer, or its legal representative, any and all such information.

_BF_   I understand the information obtained by the use of the Authorization will be used to determine eligibility for insurance, and eligibility for benefits under any existing policy. Any information obtained will not be released by/to any organization EXCEPT to the group policyholder, my employer, reinsuring companies, the Medical Information Bureau, Inc., or other persons or organizations performing business or legal services in connection with my application, claim, or as may be otherwise lawfully required or as I may further authorize.

_BF_   I further agree that a photographic copy of this Authorization shall be valid as the original. This Authorization shall be valid for one year from the date shown below.

Signature of Insured: _B. A. Fraide_   Date: _Feb. 1, 20XX_

Signature of Spouse: _Nada Fraide_   Date: _Feb. 1, 20XX_

CHS COMMUNITY HOSPITAL
9876 CLINTON AVE.
COLTER, CO 81222

Patient Name	Patient No.	Sex	Date of Birth	Admission Date	Discharge Date	Page #
DEE PENDENT	3307022	F	04/12/98	02/03/XX	02/03/XX	1

Guarantor Name and Address
CODIE PENDENT
1111 E. DUNPHY AVE
COLTER, CO 81222

Insurance Company   ROVER INSURERS, INC
Claim Number   47
Attending Physician   NOAH PULSE, M.D.

DATE OF SERVICE	DESCRIPTION OF HOSPITAL SERVICES	SERVICE CODE	QTY.	CHARGES	TOTAL CHARGES
	DETAIL OF CURRENT CHARGES				
02/03/XX	ER BASE CHARGE	40200600	1	250.00	
	** TOTAL ER SERVICES	**			250.00
02/03/XX	MIN SURG TIME 1.00HR	40200529	1	530.00	
02/03/XX	SUR-MONITR EKG CHG	40200784	1	58.00	
02/03/XX	SURG-BOVIE	40200826	1	32.00	
02/03/XX	RECOV EMERG	40202384	1	236.00	
02/03/XX	MINOR TRAY	40205049	1	116.00	
02/03/XX	PULSE OXIMETER	40205189	1	46.00	
02/03/XX	SUTURE MINOR 1-5	40205403	1	63.00	
02/03/XX	SUR-MONITR 8/P CHG	40205460	1	58.00	
02/03/XX	PACU VS MONITORING	40205635	1	75.00	
	** TOTAL SURGERY AND RECOVERY	**			1,214.00
02/03/XX	OBSERVATION ROOM	40300014	1	150.00	
	** TOTAL DAY CARE SERVICES	**			150.00
02/03/XX	NITROUS 60MIN	40404824	1	160.00	
02/03/XX	FORANE 60 MIN	40405110	1	156.00	
02/03/XX	OXYGEN 60 MIN	40405318	1	65.00	
02/03/XX	ANESTH UNIT	40405912	1	260.00	
02/03/XX	ANES 02/SENSOR	40405920	1	150.00	
	** TOTAL ANESTHESIOLOGY	**			791.00
02/03/XX	AIR WAY	40503062	1	8.50	
02/03/XX	BNDG ELASTOMULL 3 IN	40515983	1	7.50	
02/03/XX	KIT OUTPATIENT SURG	40518276	1	32.75	
02/03/XX	DRSNG GZE 4X4(10)	40525289	1	5.75	
02/03/XX	DRESS-TELFA 3X4	40525909	1	1.25	
02/03/XX	ELECTRODE DISPERS (BOVIE PAD)	40528085	1	28.50	
02/03/XX	GLOVES SURG	40532053	2	4.50	
02/03/XX	KLEENEX	40542086	1	1.25	
02/03/XX	O2 MASK	40549412	1	20.50	
02/03/XX	O2 HUMIDIFIER	40549420	1	30.25	
02/03/XX	PAC-BASIC SET UP	40550055	1	87.50	
02/03/XX	PILLOW DISP	40555252	1	12.25	
02/03/XX	SOL-IRRIGT NS 1L	40564189	1	11.00	
02/03/XX	STCKNEIT,STER 4-6	40567125	1	19.75	
02/03/XX	SUCTN FRAZIER	40569388	1	12.25	
02/03/XX	SUCTN LINER 2000	40569279	1	26.75	
02/03/XX	SUCTION YANKAUR HNDL	40569303	1	38.50	

CHS COMMUNITY HOSPITAL
9876 CLINTON AVE.
COLTER, CO 81222

Patient Name	Patient No.	Sex	Date of Birth	Admission Date	Discharge Date	Page #
DEE PENDENT	3307022	F	04/12/98	02/03/XX	02/03/XX	2

Guarantor Name and Address
CODIE PENDENT
1111 E. DUNPHY AVE
COLTER, CO 81222

Insurance Company   ROVER INSURERS, INC
Claim Number   47
Attending Physician   NOAH PULSE, M.D.

DATE OF SERVICE	DESCRIPTION OF HOSPITAL SERVICES	SERVICE CODE	QTY.	CHARGES	TOTAL CHARGES
02/03/XX	TRAY SKIN PREP W/PVP I	40577579	1	26.75	
02/03/XX	TBE CONNECTGN 120	40578189	1	14.00	
02/03/XX	PACK TOWEL (6)	40579039	1	14.00	
02/03/XX	THERMOMETER GLASS	40579096	1	4.50	
02/03/XX	URINE CUP 40580037		1	2.25	
	** TOTAL CENTRAL SUPPLY	**			
02/03/XX	PATH DIAG, SM PART-A	40705105	1	70.00	410.25
02/03/XX	PATH HANDLING PART-A	40705196	1	35.50	
	** TOTAL LAB PATH	**			
02/03/XX	ANECTINE GTTS	41742800	1	24.00	105.50
02/03/XX	PENTOTHAL SDM 1GM	41756305	1	77.50	
	** TOTAL PHARMACY	**			
02/03/XX	IV CATHETER	47136049	1	24.00	101.50
02/03/XX	IV START KIT	47137195	1	36.00	
02/03/XX	IV TUBING EXTENSION SET	47137278	1	14.00	
02/03/XX	IV TUBING PRIMARY SET	47137534	1	31.00	
02/03/XX	SOL-D-5 LR 500ML	47138169	1	44.00	
	** TOTAL IV THERAPY	**			
	SUMMARY OF CHARGES				149.00
				250.00	
	ER SERVICES			101.50	
	PHARMACY			149.00	
	IV THERAPY			858.25	
	MED-SUR SUPPLIES			105.50	
	PATHOLOGY LAB OR (PATH LAB)			530.00	
	OR SERVICES			791.00	
	ANESTHESIA			150.00	
	AMBUL SURG			236.00	
	RECOVERY ROOM				
	SUBTOTAL OF CHARGES				3,171.25
	PAYMENTS AND ADJUSTMENTS			200.00	
	SUBTOTAL PAYMENTS/ADJ				200.00
	BALANCE				2,971.25
	BALANCE DUE				2,971.25

CHS COMMUNITY HOSPITAL
9876 CLINTON AVE.
COLTER, CO 81222

Patient Name	Patient No.	Sex	Date of Birth	Admission Date	Discharge Date	Page #
RHEA ALLITY	3309176	F	11/25/90	02/01/XX	02/01/XX	1

Guarantor Name and Address

RAY ALLITY
426 KIRBY STREET
COLTON, CO 81222

Insurance Company   ROVER INSURERS, INC.
Claim Number   48

Attending Physician   WILL KUTTEROFF, M.D.

DATE OF SERVICE	DESCRIPTION OF HOSPITAL SERVICES	SERVICE CODE	QTY.	CHARGES	TOTAL CHARGES
	SUMMARY OF CHARGES				
2/01/XX	PHARMACY			100.00	
2/01/XX	IV THERAPY			151.00	
2/01/XX	MED-SURG SUPPLIES			1,237.00	
2/01/XX	PATHOLOGY LAB OR (PATH LAB)			105.50	
2/01/XX	OR SERVICES			473.00	
2/01/XX	ANESTHESIA			55.00	
2/01/XX	AMBUL SURG			150.00	
2/01/XX	RECOVERY ROOM			236.00	
	SUBTOTAL OF CHARGES				2,507.50
	PAYMENTS AND ADJUSTMENTS			NONE	
	SUBTOTAL PAYMENTS/ADJ				NONE
	BALANCE				2,507.50
	BALANCE DUE				2,507.50

CHS COMMUNITY HOSPITAL
9876 CLINTON AVE.
COLTER, CO 81222

Patient Name	Patient No.	Sex	Date of Birth	Admission Date	Discharge Date	Page #
SHERRY ATTRICKS	3309416	F	03/12/38	02/01/XX	02/01/XX	1

Guarantor Name and Address

SHERRY ATTRICKS
ROUTE 1, BOX 83
COLTER, CO 81235

Insurance Company   **BALL INS. CARRIERS**
Claim Number   49

Attending Physician   YU B. SICKMAN, M.D.

DATE OF SERVICE	DESCRIPTION OF HOSPITAL SERVICES	SERVICE CODE	QTY.	CHARGES	TOTAL CHARGES
	SUMMARY OF CHARGES				
	PHARMACY			111.50	
	IV THERAPY			171.00	
	MED-SUR SUPPLIES			1,134.25	
	PATHOLOGY LAB OR (PATH LAB)			101.00	
	OR SERVICES			630.00	
	ANESTHESIA			65.00	
	RESPIRATORY SVC			73.00	
	AMBUL SURG			150.00	
	RECOVERY ROOM			236.00	
	SUBTOTAL OF CHARGES				2,671.75
	PAYMENTS AND ADJUSTMENTS			NONE	
	SUBTOTAL PAYMENTS/ADJ				NONE
	BALANCE				2,671.75
	BALANCE DUE				2,671.75

Document 34

CHS COMMUNITY HOSPITAL
9876 CLINTON AVE.
COLTER, CO 81222

Patient Name	Patient No.	Sex	Date of Birth	Admission Date	Discharge Date	Page #
JEANETTE AKENJA-NEARING	3309416	F	10/04/72	02/25/XX	02/26/XX	1

Guarantor Name and Address

GENE POOLE (Husband)
4738 JESSUP ROAD
JASPER, CO 81335

Insurance Company   WINTER INS. CO.
Claim Number   50

Attending Physician   ALLOTA PAYNE, M.D.

FROM	THRU	ACCT CODE	DESCRIPTION	TIMES	PRICE	AMOUNT
02-25	02-25		14-01 OB/GYN ROOM	1	411.30	411.30
			TOTAL ROOM AND BOARD CHARGES	1		411.30
02-25	02-25	37210	ANTIBODY SCREEN	1	55.60	55.60
02-25	02-25	37547	BLOOD COUNT CBC	1	39.35	39.35
02-25	02-25	37731	PRO TIME	1	47.80	47.80
02-25	02-25	37733	P.T.T.	1	59.75	59.75
02-25	02-25	37742	TYPE & RH	1	58.15	58.15
02-25	02-25	37814	VDRL RPR	1	36.20	36.20
			TOTAL LABORATORY-CLINICAL			296.85
02-25	02-25	39048	AMERICAINE SPRAY	1	20.25	20.25
02-25	02-25	39106	AQUAMEP.1MG/.5ML INJ	1	11.25	11.25
02-25	02-25	41206	MASSE BREAST CRM 60G	1	30.00	30.00
02-25	02-25	41230	METHERGINE 0.2MG TAB	4	2.50	10.00
02-26	02-26	41230	METHERGINE 0.2MG TAB	4	2.50	10.00
02-25	02-25	41230	METHERGINE 0.2MG TAB	2	2.50	5.00
02-25	02-25	41504	PITOCIN 10U INJ	2	11.24	22.48
02-25	02-25	41877	TUCKS PADS #40 TOP	1	20.15	20.15
02-25	02-25	41886	TYLENOL/COD 30MG TAB	1	2.25	2.25
02-26	02-26	41886	TYLENOL/COD 30MG TAB	2	2.25	4.50
02-25	02-25	42099	ERYTHROMYCIN OPTH OINT 3.5GM	1	11.24	11.24
02-25	02-25	54092	BOTTLE PERI	1	2.85	2.85
02-25	02-25	58300	IV SOL DEXT 5% LACT RINGER 10	1	38.20	38.20
02-25	02-25	58376	IV IRRIG SOL WATER 2000 R5005	1	43.85	43.85
			TOTAL PHARMACY			232.02
02-25	02-25	50290	KIT PERSONAL COMFORT MH	1	5.85	5.85
02-25	02-25	51223	BELT SANITARY	1	10.35	10.35
02-26	02-26	51223	BELT SANITARY	1	10.35	10.35
02-25	02-25	51810	TUBING IV PRIMARY IVAC	1	16.40	16.40
02-25	02-25	51929	PACK DELIVERY VAGINAL CUSTOM	1	140.35	140.35
02-25	02-25	51935	PACK COLD ABCO	1	4.50	4.50
02-25	02-25	51961	PAD PERI STERILE PK 12	1	9.20	9.20
02-26	02-26	51961	PAD PERI STERILE PK 12	1	9.20	9.20

CHS COMMUNITY HOSPITAL
9876 CLINTON AVE.
COLTER, CO 81222

Patient Name	Patient No.	Sex	Date of Birth	Admission Date	Discharge Date	Page #
JEANETTE AKENJA-NEARING	14 52 19	F	10/04/72	02/25/XX	02/26/XX	2

Guarantor Name and Address

GENE POOLE (Husband)
4738 JESSUP ROAD
JASPER, CO 81335

Insurance Company   WINTER INS. CO.
Claim Number   49

Attending Physician   ALLOTA PAYNE, M.D.

FROM	THRU	ACCT CODE	DESCRIPTION	TIMES	PRICE	AMOUNT
02-26	02-26	51961	PAD PERI STERILE PK 12	1	9.20	9.20
02-25	02-25	52153	RAZOR DISP TOMAC	1	3.90	3.90
02-25	02-25	52173	SUCTION CATHETER CUTTER 10FR	1	3.40	3.40
02-25	02-25	52480	UNDERPADS ADULT PK 6	1	6.20	6.20
02-25	02-25	52480	UNDERPADS ADULT PK 6	1	6.20	6.20
02-25	02-25	52480	UNDERPADS ADULT PK 6	1	6.20	6.20
02-26	02-26	52480	UNDERPADS ADULT PK 6	1	6.20	6.20
02-25	02-25	52731	IV CATH QUIK (ALL SIZES)	1	13.45	13.45
02-25	02-25	52765	IV START PAK 18 11/4	1	14.65	14.65
02-25	02-25	52765	IV START PAK 18 11/4	1	14.65	14.65
02-25	02-25	53167	TRAY PREP SURGICAL EZ	1	29.90	29.90
02-25	02-25	52308	TRAY PREP SOAP/WATER	1	25.85	25.85
02-25	02-25	53254	TRAY PARACERVICAL PUDENDAL PH	1	74.20	74.20
02-25	02-25	54042	MONITOR IVAC DAILY	1	28.10	28.10
02-25	02-25	56137	AMNIHOOK MEMBRANE PERFORATOR	1	5.85	5.85
02-25	02-25	58411	GLOVE SURGICAL STERILE ALL SI	1	4.90	4.90
02-25	02-25	58411	GLOVE SURGICAL STERILE ALL SI	1	4.90	4.90
02-25	02-25	58411	GLOVE SURGICAL STERILE ALL SI	1	4.90	4.90
			TOTAL MED-SURG SUPPLIES & DEVICES	1		468.85

SUMMARY OF CHARGES

			TOTAL ROOM AND BOARD CHARGES	1		411.30
			TOTAL LABORATORY-CLINICAL			296.85
			TOTAL PHARMACY			232.02
			TOTAL MED-SURG SUPPLIES & DEVICES			468.85
			AMOUNT DUE			1,409.02

CHS COMMUNITY HOSPITAL
9876 CLINTON AVE.
COLTER, CO 81222

Patient Name	Patient No.	Sex	Date of Birth	Admission Date	Discharge Date	Page #
WADE N. POOLE	14 52 20	M	02/25/XX	02/25/XX	02/26/XX	1

Guarantor Name and Address

GENE POOLE (Father)
4738 JESSUP ROAD
JASPER, CO 81335

Insurance Company   WINTER INS. CO.
Claim Number   51

Attending Physician   ALLOTA PAYNE, M.D.

FROM	THRU	ACCT CODE	DESCRIPTION	TIMES	PRICE	AMOUNT
02-25	02-25		1400-01 NURSERY	1	240.60	240.60
			TOTAL ROOM AND BOARD CHARGES			240.60
02-26	02-26	21002	DEL RM NEWBORN SCREENING	1	41.00	41.00
			TOTAL LABOR ROOM/DELIVERY			41.00
02-26	02-26	30289	RADIOLOGY-PORTABLE STUDIES	1	51.70	51.70
02-26	02-26	30500	RADIOLOGY-SKULL, 2 VIEWS	1	95.50	95.50
			TOTAL RADIOLOGY-DIAGNOSTIC			147.20
02-25	02-25	40183	TRIPLE DYE	1	11.25	11.25
02-25	02-25	40184	VASELINE OINT 60 OZ	1	12.90	12.90
02-25	02-25	55247	WASHCLOTH BABY MOIST	1	10.80	10.80
			TOTAL PHARMACY			34.95
02-25	02-25	52481	PAMPERS NEWBORN	1	16.10	16.10
			TOTAL MED-SURG SUPPLIES & DEVICES			16.10
			SUMMARY OF CHARGES			
			TOTAL ROOM AND BOARD CHARGES	1		240.60
			TOTAL LABOR ROOM/DELIVERY			41.00
			TOTAL RADIOLOGY-DIAGNOSTIC			147.20
			TOTAL PHARMACY			34.95
			TOTAL MED/SURG SUPPLIES & DEVICES			16.10
			AMOUNT DUE			479.85

ROVER INSURERS, INC.
5931 ROLLING ROAD
RONSON, CO 81369

PATIENT NAME	DATE OF SERVICE	PROCEDURE	BILLED AMOUNT	ALLOWED AMOUNT	% OF AMOUNT	PAYMENT AMOUNT	DENIED AMOUNT	REASON CODE
PENDENT, CODIE	01/17/XX	IND PSYCH	$160.00	$112.50	80%	$ 0.00*	$ 47.50	36
	01/17/XX	PSYCH TESTING	$575.00	$ 0.00		$ 0.00	$575.00	91
	TOTAL		$735.00	$112.50		$ 0.00	$622.50	
ALLITY, MORT	01/17/XX	HEM PLAT/DIF	$ 11.00	$ 5.00	80%	$ 4.00	$ 6.00	36
	01/17/XX	CPK	$ 56.00	$ 56.00	80%	$ 44.80	$ 0.00	36
	01/17/XX	AMYLASE	$ 19.00	$ 9.00	80%	$ 7.20	$ 10.00	36
	01/17/XX	COMP MET PAN	$130.00	$ 76.00	80%	$ 60.80	$ 54.00	36
	01/18/XX	LDH	$ 16.00	$ 6.00	80%	$ 4.80	$ 10.00	36
	TOTAL		$232.00	$152.00		$121.60	$ 80.00	
TOTALS			**$967.00**	**$264.50**		**$121.60**	**$702.50**	

REASON CODES:

36 BILLED AMOUNT EXCEEDS AMOUNT ALLOWED BY THE PLAN.
91 PSYCHOLOGICAL TESTING IS NOT COVERED BY YOUR PLAN.
*   APPLIED TOWARD DEDUCTIBLE

DETACH CHECK BEFORE CASHING

ROVER INSURERS, INC.
5931 ROLLING ROAD
RONSON, CO 81369

BANK OF COLORS (970) 555-5555   04-10345
Ronson Branch
2300 Rocky Road   08-12
Ronson, CO 81369   1100

                                    February 28,   20 XX $ 121.60

PAY   One Hundred Twenty One and 60/100** DOLLARS

TO
THE   Consolidated Health Services
ORDER   1357 Castle Blvd, Suite 515
OF   Colter, CO 81222-2222   *Randy Rover*
                                                       ‖0000011123‖0

‖0001111‖0 ⑆111000123⑆: 0123 4567‖0

BALL INSURANCE CARRIERS
3895 BUBBLE BLVD.
BOXWOOD, CO 85926

PATIENT NAME	DATE OF SERVICE	PROCEDURE	BILLED AMOUNT	ALLOWED AMOUNT	BASIC AMOUNT	80 % AMOUNT	DENIED AMOUNT	REASON CODE
FEVER, TY PHOID	01/21/XX	OFFICE VISIT	$150.00	$117.50	6.75	$ 0.00*	$ 32.50	19
	TOTAL		$150.00	$117.50	6.75	$ 0.00	$ 32.50	
TIRED, BARRY	01/21/XX	OFFICE VISIT	$190.00	$148.00	8.50	$ 11.60*	$ 42.00	19
	01/21/XX	CBC	$ 30.00	$ 15.00	.75	$ 11.40	$ 15.00	19
	01/21/XX	HIV I & II	$ 30.00	$ 21.00	1.11	$ 15.91	$ 9.00	19
	01/21/XX	HEPATITIS B	$ 30.00	$ 21.00	1.11	$ 15.91	$ 9.00	19
	01/21/XX	T CELL COUNT	$ 30.00	$ 9.00	.50	$ 6.80	$ 21.00	19
	TOTAL		$310.00	$214.00	11.97	$ 61.62	$ 96.00	
TOTALS			**$460.00**	**$331.50**	**18.72**	**$ 61.62**	**$128.50**	

REASON CODES:

19   BILLED AMOUNT EXCEEDS AMOUNT ALLOWED BY THE PLAN.
*   APPLIED TOWARD DEDUCTIBLE

DETACH CHECK BEFORE CASHING

BALL INSURANCE CARRIERS
3895 BUBBLE BLVD.
BOXWOOD, CO 85926

BANK OF COLORS (970) 555-5555
Boxwood Branch
2300 Barker Blvd.
Boxwood, CO 85926

2345

01-11 / 1000

February 21,   20 XX

PAY   Eighty and 34/100   DOLLARS $ 80.34

TO THE ORDER OF   Consolidated Health Services
1357 Castle Blvd, Suite 515
Colter, CO 81222-2222

Bob Brader

||□001111||□ |:111000123|:   0123   4567||□ ||□000011123||□

WINTER INSURANCE
9763 WESTERN WAY
WHITTIER, CO 82963

PATIENT NAME	DATE OF SERVICE	PROCEDURE	BILLED AMOUNT	ALLOWED AMOUNT	% OF AMOUNT	PAYMENT AMOUNT	DENIED AMOUNT	REASON CODE
POOLE, CARLA	01/14/XX	OFFICE VISIT	$ 85.00	$ 55.00	100%*	$ 55.00	$ 30.00	45
	01/14/XX	X-RAY FINGER	$ 40.00	$ 31.00	100%*	$ 31.00	$ 9.00	45
	01/14/XX	STERILE TRAY	$ 50.00	$ 50.00	100%*	$ 50.00	$ 0.00	45
	TOTAL		$175.00	$136.00		$136.00	$ 39.00	

AKENJA-NEARING, JEANETTE   PENDED (ALL PRE- AND POST-PARTUM CARE CHARGES ARE INCLUDED IN LABOR AND DELIVERY CHARGE)

| TOTALS | | | $175.00 | $136.00 | | $136.00 | $ 39.00 | |

REASON CODES:

45   BILLED AMOUNT EXCEEDS AMOUNT ALLOWED BY THE PLAN.
*   ACCIDENT BENEFIT AMOUNT

DETACH CHECK BEFORE CASHING

WINTER INSURANCE
9763 WESTERN WAY
WHITTIER, CO 82963

BANK OF COLORS
Whittier Branch
2300 Whyme Way
Whittier, CO 82963

(970) 555-5555

04-9999
33-77
1293

February 26,   20 XX $ 136.00

PAY   One Hundred Thirty Six and 00/100**   DOLLARS $ 136.00

TO
THE
ORDER
OF

Consolidated Health Services
1357 Castle Blvd, Suite 515
Colter, CO 81222-2222

Tom Trustee

⑈001111⑈ ⑆111000123⑆: 0123 4567⑈⑉ ⑈0000011123⑈⑉

Document 39

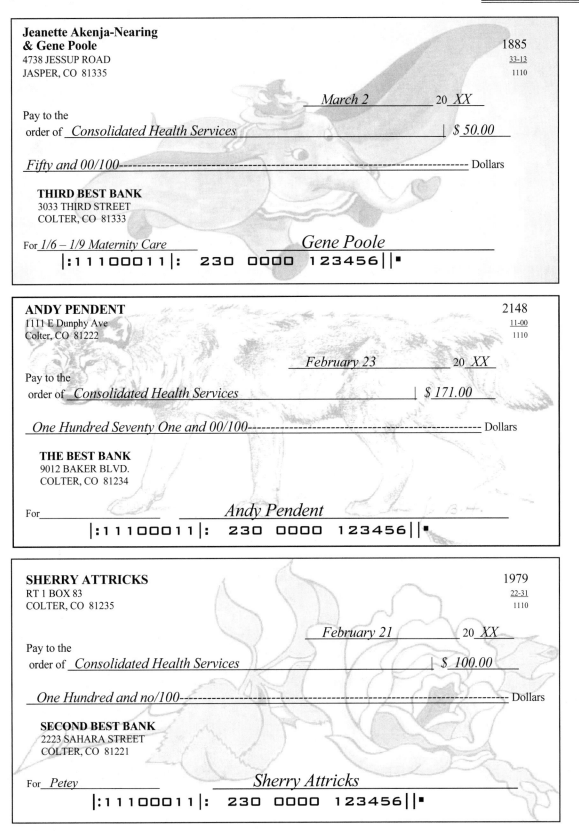

Jeanette Akenja-Nearing
& Gene Poole 1885
4738 JESSUP ROAD 33-13
JASPER, CO 81335 1110

March 2 20 *XX*

Pay to the
order of *Consolidated Health Services* | $ *50.00*

Fifty and 00/100-- Dollars

THIRD BEST BANK
3033 THIRD STREET
COLTER, CO 81333

For *1/6 – 1/9 Maternity Care* *Gene Poole*

|:11100011|: 230 0000 123456||▪

ANDY PENDENT 2148
1111 E Dunphy Ave 11-00
Colter, CO 81222 1110

February 23 20 *XX*

Pay to the
order of *Consolidated Health Services* | $ *171.00*

One Hundred Seventy One and 00/100-- Dollars

THE BEST BANK
9012 BAKER BLVD.
COLTER, CO 81234

For *Andy Pendent*

|:11100011|: 230 0000 123456||▪

SHERRY ATTRICKS 1979
RT 1 BOX 83 22-31
COLTER, CO 81235 1110

February 21 20 *XX*

Pay to the
order of *Consolidated Health Services* | $ *100.00*

One Hundred and no/100-- Dollars

SECOND BEST BANK
2223 SAHARA STREET
COLTER, CO 81221

For *Petey* *Sherry Attricks*

|:11100011|: 230 0000 123456||▪

Document 39

Ray Allity   918
426 Kirby Street   11-00
Colton, CO 81223   1110

March 2,   20 *XX*

Pay to the
order of *Consolidated Health Services* | $ *100.00*

One Hundred and 00/100-- Dollars

THE BEST BANK
9012 BAKER BLVD.
COLTER, CO 81234

For   *Ray Allity*

|:11100011|: 230 0000 123456||⑃

KENT C. & JUANA FORE-THEROAD   1195
9871 INDUSTRIAL ROAD   11-00
COLTER, CO 81222   1110

February 23,   20 *XX*

Pay to the
order of *Consolidated Health Services* | $ *60.00*

Sixty and 00/100--Dollars

THE BEST BANK
9012 BAKER BLVD.
COLTER, CO 81234

For   *Kent C. Theroad*

|:11100011|: 230 0000 123456||⑃

ER REPORTS

On 2/9/XX the Theroad family was involved in an auto accident. They were traveling in the rain about 8 a.m., going west on Interstate 70 near the Island Blvd. exit in Inglewood, CO. The car in front of them lost control and turned sideways. Juana Fore-Theroad was driving. She successfully attempted to avoid the other car, but lost control. The Theroad car slid, flipped over the guardrail, and rolled several times down a steep embankment. Due to the severity of injuries, the family was transported to CHS Community Hospital where they were treated by several doctors in the ER.

CLAIM 54
Juana Fore-Theroad was seen in the hospital on 2/9/XX by Dr. Butch M. N. Hackim. She received a comprehensive history and exam visit in the emergency room ($240). Juana was not wearing her seat belt and her face struck the steering wheel. The hospital took complete x-rays of the facial bones (3 views) ($50), skull (5 views w/o stereo) ($85), and cervical spine ($40), which Dr. Hackim interpreted. Diagnosis: shock, fracture of the nose, depression fracture of the zygomatic arch, puncture wound to the lower right jaw bone with embedded 1 cm. foreign body (jaw fractured), multiple contusions and lacerations of the facial area, concussion. Juana was promptly admitted to the ICU for stabilization and observation prior to surgery.

CLAIM 55
Kent C. Theroad was in the front passenger seat and was wearing his seat belt. Dr. Noah Pulse, the ER doctor, performed a detailed history and exam in the emergency room ($150). Patient complained of pain in the left arm and x-rays (ulna, 3 views) were performed by the hospital technician, which Dr. Pulse interpreted ($30). Diagnosis: Broken medial ulna and mild shock. Dr. Pulse was unable to cast the arm due to swelling, so a splint was applied and Kent was admitted for observation.

CLAIM 56
Ian N. Theroad was in the back seat. He was not wearing his seat belt and was thrown from the car. The car rolled over when he was partially extended, crushing his right leg. After becoming dislodged, he rolled several times down the hill, striking his head. He was unconscious and on advanced life support when brought into the emergency room. He received critical care for two hours in the emergency department ($600), along with an MRI of the right thigh ($700), and x-rays of the skull (6 views) ($85), full spine a and p ($100), right leg (a/p & lat of femur and tibia/fibula) ($65 ea), left leg (a/p & lat of femur and tibia/fibula) ($65 each), and both arms (a/p & lat of both upper and lower rt and lt arm) ($65 each). Diagnosis: shock, crushing injury to right thigh with multiple open fractures of the right leg, skull fracture with brain swelling, cervical spinal injuries. Treatment was performed by Dr. Kent Cure, M.D., who also directed the treatment of the EMS personnel while they were treating Ian and Juana ($75 each).

CLAIM 57
Donette Theroad was in her car seat and was asleep at the time of the accident. Although scared and bruised, she appeared to suffer no major injuries. However, an expanded problem-focused exam of low complexity ($45) was performed by Dr. Noah Pulse. Diagnosis: auto accident, multiple contusions. She was released to the care of her aunt.

[Carrier] Summer Insurance Company
CONTRACT HOLDER: Rocky Company

SMALL GROUP HMO CONTRACT
EFFECTIVE DATE OF CONTRACT:
January 1, 1998

ELIGIBILITY

Employees: Actively at work for a minimum of 35 hours per week. Is eligible after 30 continuous work days.

Employee's who enroll more than 30 days after their employment date are considered Late Enrollees. Late Enrollees are subject to this Contract's Pre-existing Conditions limitation.

Coverage terminates the date an Employee ceases to be an Actively at Work, Full-Time Employee for any reason.

Dependents: Dependents include the Employee's legal spouse, the Employee's unmarried Dependent children who are under age 19, and the Employee's unmarried Dependent children, from age 19 until their 23rd birthday, who are enrolled as full-time students at accredited schools.

Exception: Any dependent who does not reside in the Service Area is not an eligible Dependent. Eligible Dependents will not include any Dependent who is covered by this Contract as an Employee or on active duty in the armed forces of any country.

"Unmarried Dependent children" include legally adopted children, step-children if they depend on the Employee for most of their support and maintenance and children under a court appointed guardianship.

THE ROLE OF A MEMBER'S PRIMARY CARE PHYSICIAN (PCP)

A Member's PCP provides basic health maintenance services and coordinates a Member's overall health care. Anytime a Member needs medical care, the Member should contact his or her Primary Care Physician. In a Medical Emergency, a Member may go directly to the emergency room. If a Member does, then the Member must call his or her Primary Care Physician or the Care Manager and Member Services within 48 hours, or We will provide services under this HMO Plan only if We determine that notice was given as soon as was reasonably possible.

REFERRAL FORMS

A Member can be referred for Specialist Services by a Member's PCP. Except in the case of a Medical Emergency, a Member will not be eligible for any services provided by anyone other than a Member's PCP (including but not limited to Specialist Services) if a Member has not been referred by his or her PCP. Referrals must be obtained prior to receiving services and supplies from any Practitioner other than the Member's PCP.

MEDICAL NECESSITY

Members will receive designated benefits only when Medically Necessary and Appropriate. We or the Care Manager may determine whether any benefit was Medically Necessary and Appropriate, and We have the option to select the appropriate Participating Hospital to render services if hospitalization is necessary. Decisions as to what is Medically Necessary and Appropriate are subject to review by our quality assessment committee or its physician designee.

LIMITATION ON SERVICES

Except in cases of Medical Emergency, services are available only from Participating Providers. We shall have no liability or obligation to cover any service or benefit sought or received by a Member from any Physician, Hospital, other Provider unless prior arrangements are made by us.

SCHEDULE OF SERVICES AND SUPPLIES

The services or supplies covered under the contract are subject to all copayments and are determined per calendar year per Member, unless otherwise stated. Maximums apply only to the specific services provided.

SERVICES COPAYMENTS: Copayment $15, unless otherwise stated

Emergency Room Copayment $50, credited toward Inpatient admission if admitted within 24 hours

Coinsurance 0% except as stated on the Schedule of Services and Supplies for Prescription Drugs

MAXIMUM LIFETIME BENEFITS Unlimited, **except** as otherwise stated

HOSPITAL SERVICES:

Inpatient $150 Copayment/day for a maximum of 5 days/admission. Maximum Copayment $1,500/Calendar Year. Unlimited days.

Outpatient $15 Copayment/visit

PRACTITIONER SERVICES RECEIVED AT A HOSPITAL:

Inpatient Visit $0 Copayment

Outpatient Visit $15 Copayment/visit; no Copayment if any other Copayment applies.

Emergency Room $50 Copayment/visit/Member (credited toward Inpatient Admission if Admission occurs within 24 hours)

SURGERY:

Inpatient $0 Copayment

Outpatient $15 Copayment/visit

HOME HEALTH CARE Unlimited days, if preapproved; $0 Copayment.

HOSPICE SERVICES Unlimited days, if preapproved; $0 Copayment.

MATERNITY/PRENATAL CARE $25 Copayment for initial visit only; $0 Copayment thereafter.

MENTAL NERVOUS CONDITIONS AND SUBSTANCE ABUSE:

Outpatient $15 Copayment/visit maximum 20 visits/Calendar Year.

Inpatient $150 Copayment/day for a maximum of 5 days per admission. Maximum Copayment: $1,500/Calendar Year. Maximum of 30 days inpatient care/Calendar Year. One Inpatient day may be exchanged for two Outpatient visits.

THERAPEUTIC MANIPULATION $15 Copayment/visit; maximum 30 visits/Calendar Year

PODIATRIC $15 Copayment/visit (excludes Routine Foot Care).

PREADMISSION TESTING $15 Copayment/visit.

PRESCRIPTION DRUG 50% Coinsurance [May be substituted by Carrier with $15 Copayment.]

PRIMARY CARE PHYSICIAN $15 Copayment/visit.

OR CARE MANAGER SERVICES (OUTSIDE HOSPITAL)

PRIMARY CARE SERVICES $15 Copayment/visit.

REHABILITATION SERVICES Subject to the Inpatient Hospital Services Copayment above. The Copayment does not apply if Admission is immediately preceded by a Hospital Inpatient Stay.

SECOND SURGICAL OPINION $15 Copayment/visit.

SPECIALIST SERVICES $15 Copayment/visit.

SKILLED NURSING CENTER Unlimited days, if preapproved; $0 Copayment.

THERAPY SERVICES $15 Copayment/visit.

DIAGNOSTIC SERVICES .

INPATIENT $0 Copayment

OUTPATIENT $15 Copayment/visit

NOTE: No services or supplies will be provided if a Member fails to obtain pre-authorization of care through his or her primary care physician or health center or care manager. Read the Member provisions carefully before obtaining medical care, services or supplies. Refer to the section of this contract called "Noncovered Services and Supplies" for a list of the services and supplies for which a Member is not eligible for coverage under this contract.

COVERED SERVICES & SUPPLIES

Under this HMO Plan, Members are entitled to receive the benefits in the following sections when Medically Necessary and Appropriate, subject to the payment by Members of applicable copayments as stated in the applicable Schedule of Services and Supplies.

(a) **OUTPATIENT SERVICES.** The following services are covered only at the PCP's office, or elsewhere upon prior written Referral by a Member's PCP:

1. **Office visits** during office hours, and during non-office hours when medically necessary.
2. **Home visits** by a Member's PCP.
3. **Periodic health examinations** to include:
   a. Well child care from birth including immunizations;
   b. Routine physical examinations, including eye examinations;
   c. Routine gynecologic exams and related services;
   d. Routine ear and hearing examination; and
   e. Routine allergy injections and immunizations (but not if solely for the purpose of travel or as a requirement of a Member's employment).
4. **Diagnostic Services**.
5. **Casts and dressings.**
6. **Ambulance Service** when certified in writing as Medically Necessary by a Member's PCP and approved in advance by us.
7. **Procedures and prescription drugs to enhance fertility,** except where specifically excluded in this Contract.
8. **Prosthetic Devices** when we arrange for them. We cover only the initial fitting and purchase of artificial limbs and eyes, and other prosthetic devices. We do not cover replacements, repairs, wigs.
9. **Durable Medical Equipment** when ordered by a Member's PCP and arranged through us.
10. **Prescription Drugs and contraceptives which require a Practitioner's prescription**, insulin syringes and needles, glucose test strips and lancets, colostomy bags, belts and irrigators when obtained through a Participating Provider. A prescription or refill will not include more than:
    a. the greater of a 30 day supply or 100 unit doses for each prescription or refill; or
    b. the amount usually prescribed by the Member's Participating Provider.
11. **Nutritional Counseling** for the management of disease.
12. **Dental x-rays** when related to Covered Services.
13. **Oral surgery** in connection with bone fractures, removal of tumors and orthodontogenic cysts, and other surgical procedures, as we approve.
14. **Food and Food Products for Inherited Metabolic Diseases**: We cover charges incurred for the therapeutic treatment of inherited metabolic diseases, including the purchase of medical foods (enteral formula) and low protein modified food products. For the purpose of this benefit: "inherited metabolic disease" means a disease caused by an inherited abnormality of body chemistry for which testing is mandated by law.

(b) **INPATIENT HOSPICE, HOSPITAL, REHABILITATION CENTER & SKILLED NURSING CENTER BENEFITS**. The following services are covered when hospitalized by a Participating Provider at Participating Hospitals (or at Nonparticipating facilities upon prior written authorization by Us):

1. Semi-private room and board accommodations except as stated below, we provide coverage for Inpatient care for:
   a. a minimum of 72 hours following a modified radical mastectomy; and
   b. a minimum of 48 hours following a simple mastectomy.

   We also provide coverage for the mother and newly born child for:
   a. up to 48 hours of inpatient care following a vaginal delivery; and
   b. a minimum of 96 hours of inpatient care following a cesarean section.

   We provide such coverage subject to the following:
   a. the attending Practitioner must determine that inpatient care is medically necessary; or
   b. the mother must request the inpatient care.
2. Private accommodations will be provided only when approved in advance by Us. If a Member occupies a private room without such certification Member shall be liable for the difference between payment by Us to the Provider and the private room rate.
3. General nursing care
4. Use of intensive or special care facilities
5. X-ray examinations including CAT scans but not dental x-rays
6. Use of operating room and related facilities
7. Magnetic resonance imaging "MRI"
8. Drugs, medications, biologicals
9. Cardiography/Encephalography
10. Laboratory testing and services
11. Pre- and postoperative care
12. Special tests
13. Nuclear medicine
14. Therapy Services
15. Oxygen and oxygen therapy
16. Anesthesia and anesthesia services
17. Blood, blood products and blood processing
18. Intravenous injections and solutions
19. Surgical, medical and obstetrical services; We also cover reconstructive breast Surgery, Surgery to restore and achieve symmetry between the two breasts and the cost of prostheses following a mastectomy on one breast or both breasts.
20. Private duty nursing only when approved in advance by us.
21. The following transplants: Cornea, Kidney, Lung, Liver, Heart and Pancreas.
22. Allogenic bone marrow transplants.
23. Autologous bone marrow transplants and associated dose intensive chemotherapy: only for treatment of Leukemia, Lymphoma, Neuroblastoma, Aplastic Anemia, Genetic Disorders (SCID and WISCOT Alldrich) and Breast Cancer, when approved in advance by Us, if the Member is participating in a clinical trial.
24. Peripheral Blood Stem Cell Transplants.

(c) **BENEFITS FOR SUBSTANCE ABUSE AND NON-BIOLOGICALLY-BASED MENTAL ILLNESSES.** The following Services are covered when rendered by a Participating Provider at Provider's office or at a Participating Substance Abuse Center or Health Center upon prior written referral by a Member's PCP. This section does *not* address coverage for a Biologically-based Mental Illness.

1. **Outpatient.** Members are entitled to receive up to twenty (20) outpatient visits per Calendar Year. Benefits include diagnosis, medical, psychiatric and psychological treatment and medical referral services by a Member's PCP or the Care Manager for the abuse of or addiction to drugs and Non-Biologically-based Mental Illnesses. Payment for non-medical ancillary services (such as vocational rehabilitation or employment counseling) is not provided. Members are additionally eligible, upon referral by a Member's PCP or the Care Manager, for up to sixty (60) more outpatient visits by exchanging one or more of the inpatient hospital days described below where each exchanged inpatient day provides two outpatient visits.
2. **Inpatient Hospital Care.** Members are entitled to receive up to thirty (30) days of inpatient care benefits for detoxification, medical treatment for medical conditions resulting from the substance abuse, referral services for substance abuse or addiction, and Non-Biologically-based Mental Illnesses.

(d) **BENEFITS FOR BIOLOGICALLY-BASED MENTAL ILLNESS OR ALCOHOL ABUSE.** We cover treatment of a Biologically-based Mental Illness or Alcohol Abuse the same way We would for any other illness. We do not pay for Custodial care, education or training.

(e) **EMERGENCY CARE BENEFITS - WITHIN AND OUTSIDE OUR SERVICE AREA.** The following Services are covered under this HMO Plan without prior written referral by a Member's PCP in the event of a Medical Emergency as Determined by Us.

1. A Member's PCP is required to provide or arrange for on-call coverage twenty-four (24) hours a day, seven (7) days a week. Unless a delay would be detrimental to a Member's health, Member shall call a Member's PCP or Health Center or Us or the

Care Manager prior to seeking emergency treatment.

2. In the event Members are hospitalized in a Nonparticipating Facility, coverage will only be provided until Members are medically able to travel or be transported to a Participating Facility. If Members elect to continue treatment with Nonparticipating Providers, We shall have no responsibility for payment beyond the date Members are Determined to be medically able to be transported. If transportation is Medically Necessary, We will cover the reasonable and customary cost. Members will be subject to all Copayments which would have been required had similar benefits been provided upon prior written referral to a Participating Provider.

3. The Copayment for an emergency room visit will be credited toward the Hospital Inpatient Copayment if Members are admitted as an Inpatient to the Hospital as a result of the Medical Emergency.

(f) **THERAPY SERVICES.** The following Services are covered.

1. Speech, Physical, Occupational, and Cognitive Therapies are covered for non-chronic conditions and acute Illnesses and Injuries. This benefit consists of treatment for a 60 day period per incident of Illness or Injury, beginning with the first day of treatment, provided that a Member's PCP certifies in writing that the treatment will result in a significant improvement of a Member's condition within this time period and treatment is approved in writing by Us.

2. Chelation Therapy, Chemotherapy treatment, Dialysis Treatment, Infusion Therapy, Radiation Therapy, and Respiration Therapy.

(g) **HOME HEALTH SERVICES.** The following Services are covered.

1. **Skilled nursing services**, provided by or under the supervision of a registered professional nurse.

2. Services of a **home health aide**, under the supervision of a registered professional nurse, or if appropriate, a qualified speech or physical therapist.

3. **Medical Social Services** by or under the supervision of a qualified medical or psychiatric social worker, in conjunction with other Home Health Services, if the PCP certifies that such services are essential for the effective treatment of a Member's medical condition.

4. **Therapy Services** as set forth above.

5. **Hospice Care** if Members are terminally Ill or terminally injured with life expectancy of six months or less, as certified by the Member's PCP. Services may include home and hospital visits by nurses and social workers; pain management and symptom control; instruction and supervision of family Members, inpatient care; counseling and emotional support; and other Home Health benefits listed above.

Nothing in this section shall require us to provide Home Health Benefits when in Our Determination the treatment setting is not appropriate, or when there is a more cost effective setting in which to provide Medically Necessary and Appropriate care.

(h) **DENTAL CARE AND TREATMENT.** The following services are covered when rendered by a Participating Practitioner upon prior Referral by a Member's PCP. We cover:

1. the diagnosis and treatment of oral tumors and cysts; and

2. the surgical removal of bony impacted teeth.
   We also cover treatment of an Injury to natural teeth or the jaw, but only if:

3. the Injury occurs while the Member is covered under any health benefit plan;

4. the Injury was not caused, directly or indirectly by biting or chewing; and

5. all treatment is finished within 6 months of the date of the Injury.
   Treatment includes replacing natural teeth lost due to such Injury. But in no event do we cover orthodontic treatment.
   For a Member who is severely disabled or who is a Child under age 6, we cover:

a. general anesthesia and Hospitalization for dental services; and

b. dental services rendered by a dentist regardless of where the dental services are provided for a medical condition covered by this Contract which requires Hospitalization or general anesthesia.

(i) **TREATMENT FOR TEMPOROMANDIBULAR JOINT DISORDER (TMJ)** Not covered. We do not cover any services or supplies for orthodontia, crowns or bridgework.

(j) **THERAPEUTIC MANIPULATION** Limited to 30 visits per Calendar Year, and no more than two modalities per visit.

NONCOVERED SERVICES AND SUPPLIES
THE FOLLOWING ARE NOT COVERED SERVICES UNDER THIS CONTRACT.
Acupuncture except when used as a substitute for other forms of anesthesia.
Ambulance services for transportation from a Hospital or other health care Facility, unless Member is being transferred to another Inpatient health care Facility.
Broken Appointments (Charges for)
Blood or blood plasma which is replaced by or for a Member.
Care and/or treatment by a **Christian Science Practitioner**.

Completion of claim forms.

Cosmetic Surgery, except as otherwise stated in this Contract; complications of Cosmetic Surgery; drugs prescribed for cosmetic purposes.

Custodial or **domiciliary** care.

Dental care or treatment, including appliances, except as otherwise stated in this Contract.

Dose intensive chemotherapy, except as otherwise stated in this Contract.

Educational services and supplies providing: training in the activities of daily living; instruction in scholastic skills such as reading and writing; preparation for an occupation; or treatment for learning disabilities.

Experimental or **Investigational** treatments, procedures, hospitalizations, drugs, biological products or medical devices, except as otherwise stated in this Contract.

Extraction of teeth, except for bony impacted teeth. Services or supplies for or in connection with:

    a. except as otherwise stated in this Contract, exams to determine the need for (or changes of) **eyeglasses** or lenses of any type;

    b. eyeglasses or lenses of any type except initial replacements for loss of the natural lens; or

    c. eye surgery such as radial keratotomy, when the primary purpose is to correct myopia (nearsightedness), hyperopia (farsightedness) or astigmatism (blurring).

Services or supplies provided by Members of the Employee's **family**.

Fertility treatments including harvesting, storage and / or manipulation of eggs and sperm. This includes, but is not limited to: in vitro fertilization; embryo transfer; embryo freezing; and Gamete intra-fallopian Transfer (GIFT) and Zygote Intrafallopian Transfer (ZIFT), drugs and drug therapy.

Hearing aids and hearing examinations to determine the need for hearing aids or the need to adjust them.

Herbal medicine.

Hypnotism.

Illegal occupations or activities.

Work-related Illness or Injury, including a condition which is the result of disease or bodily infirmity, which occurred on the job and which is covered or could have been covered for benefits provided under workers' compensation.

Local anesthesia charges.

Membership costs for health clubs, weight loss clinics and similar programs.

Marriage, career or financial counseling, sex therapy or family therapy, and related services.

Methadone maintenance.

Nonprescription drugs or supplies, except;

    a. insulin needles and syringes and glucose test strips and lancets;

    b. colostomy bags, belts, and irrigators; and

    c. as stated in this Contract for food and food products for inherited metabolic diseases.

Pastoral counseling services.

Personal convenience or comfort items.

Any service provided without prior written Referral by the Member's **PCP**, except as specified in this Contract. In the event of a Medical Emergency, any amount which is greater than the amount We Determine to be the **reasonable and customary charge**.

Rest or convalescent cures.

Room and board charges for any period of time during which the member was not physically present overnight in the Facility.

Routine Foot Care, except:

    a. an open cutting operation to treat weak, strained, flat, unstable or unbalanced feet, metatarsalgia or bunions;

    b. the removal of nail roots; and

    c. treatment or removal of corns, calluses or toenails in conjunction with the treatment of metabolic or peripheral vascular disease.

Self-administered services such as: biofeedback, patient-controlled analgesia on an Outpatient basis, related diagnostic testing, self-care and self-help training.

Services or supplies:

    a. eligible for payment under either federal or state programs (except Medicaid and Medicare);

    b. for which a charge is not usually made;

    c. for which a Member would not have been charged if he or she did not have health care coverage;

    d. provided by or in a Government Hospital unless the services are for treatment:

        • of a nonservice Medical Emergency; or

        • by a Veterans' Administration Hospital of a non-service related Illness or Injury.

Sterilization reversal.

Sex-alteration treatment, including surgery, sex hormones, and related medical, psychological and psychiatric services; services and supplies arising from complications of sex transformation.

Telephone consultations.

Transplants, except as otherwise listed in the Contract.

Transportation.

Vision therapy.

Vitamins and dietary supplements.

Services or supplies received as a result of a **war**, declared or undeclared; police actions; services in the armed forces; or riots or insurrection.

Weight reduction or control, unless there is a diagnosis of morbid obesity; special foods, food supplements, liquid diets, diet plans or any related products.

Wigs, toupees, hair transplants, hair weaving or any drug if such drug is used in connection with baldness.

COORDINATION OF BENEFITS AND SERVICES: OBD rules apply for coordination of benefits.

HMO Responsibility Form

Covered Services	MEDICARE		COMMERCIAL						
	Standard	Medi-Medi	AMG	Rocky	CAT	MIPC	CAIT	SBA	RICE
Hospital visits (99221-99239)	G	G	G	G	G	G	G	G	G
Office Visits (99201-99215)	–	G	G	G	G	G	G	G	G
Emergency department visits (99281-99285)	G	G	P	G	G	P	G	P	G
X-rays & Ultrasounds	G	G	G	G	G	G	G	G	G
Magnetic resonance imaging services	P	P	G	G	P	G	P	G	P
Lab Fees (80001-89999)	G	G	G	G	G	G	G	G	G
Inpatient surgery									
Facility charges	P	P	P	P	P	P	P	P	P
Physician visits	G	G	G	G	G	G	G	G	G
Surgeon	P	P	G	G	P	G	G	G	G
Assistant surgeon	P	P	G	G	P	G	G	G	G
Anesthesiologist	P	P	P	P	P	P	P	P	P
X-ray technician	P	P	P	P	P	P	P	P	P
Outpatient surgery									
Facility charges	P	P	P	P	P	P	P	P	P
Physician visits	G	G	G	G	G	G	G	G	G
Surgeon	P	P	G	G	P	G	G	G	G
Assistant surgeon	P	P	G	G	P	G	G	G	G
Anesthesiologist	P	P	P	P	P	P	P	P	P
X-ray technician	P	P	P	P	P	P	P	P	P

Legend: G = Medical Group Responsibility; P = Plan/HMO Responsibility; G/P = Shared Responsibility; - = Not Covered
This chart shows a sampling of CPT codes and the party that bears responsibility for covering costs for each procedure under numerous different plans. It is important to check the correct column for the plan being processed to determine if services are covered or not.

Document 42

EXPLANATION OF MEDICARE BENEFITS

DATE: FEBRUARY 27, 20XX
CHECK SEQUENCE NO.: 2AF-01241351-2
PAGE 1 OF 1

BENEFICIARY NAME HIC NO EX NO	SVC FR MO-DY	TO DY-YR	PLACE TYPE	PROCEDURE DESCRIPTION	AMOUNT BILLED	AMOUNT APPROVED	SEE NOTE	DEDUCTIBLE	COINSUR.	PAYMENT	INTEREST
PHILLIP D. CUPP	01-11	11-XX	1	DIALYSIS	115.00	96.87	56				
	01-14	14-XX	1	DIALYSIS	115.00	96.87	56				
3323568515356				TOTALS	230.00	193.74	442	100.00	18.75	74.99	0.00
PHILLIP D. CUPP	01-17	17-XX	1	DIALYSIS	115.00	96.87	56				
	01-22	22-XX	1	DIALYSIS	115.00	96.87	56				
	01-25	25-XX	1	DIALYSIS	115.00	96.87	56				
	01-27	07-XX	1	DIALYSIS	115.00	96.87	56				
3351453844				TOTALS	460.00	387.48	442	0.00	77.50	309.98	0.00
HICK CUPP	01-17	17-XX	1	VIS FLD TST	110.00	87.98	56				
	01-18	18-XX	1	EYE EXAM	205.00	159.56	56				
				TOTALS	315.00	247.54	442	100.00	0.00	0.00	0.00
BROOKE N. HART	01-06	06-XX	1	ER VISIT	195.00	161.00	56				
	01-06	06-XX	1	EKG	40.00	38.39	56				
	01-06	06-XX	1	TREADMILL	170.00	156.35	56				
	01-06	06-XX	1	CBC/PLAT	50.00	37.70	56				
	01-06	06-XX	1	THYROID	50.00	26.81	56				
	01-06	06-XX	1	HEPATIC PANEL	45.00	12.18	56				
*				TOTALS	550.00	432.43	442	100.00	29.51	118.03	0.00
BROOKE N. HART	01-07	07-XX	1	HOSP VST	250.00	219.18	56				
	01-08	08-XX	1	BL TYP/RH	35.00	14.63	56				
	01-08	08-XX	1	ABG PA	75.00	52.64	56				
	01-08	08-XX	1	R/L HT CATH	4065.00	2998.21	56				
*				TOTALS	4425.00	3284.66	442	00.00	656.93	2627.73	0.00
SHAY KEE HART	01-21	21-XX	1	OV	190.00	176.55	56				
	01-21	21-XX	1	URINALYSIS	30.00	9.91	56				
*				TOTALS	220.00	186.46	442	100.00	17.29	69.17	0.00
SHAY KEE HART	01-28	28-XX	1	PHYS THER	135.00	86.82	56				
	01-28	28-XX	1	WHIRLPOOL	25.00	19.91	56				
	01-28	28-XX	1	TRACTION N/D	25.00	18.63	56				
	02-04	04-XX	1	PHYS THER	135.00	86.82	56				
	02-04	04-XX	1	WHIRLPOOL	25.00	19.91	56				
	02-04	04-XX	1	TRACTION N/D	25.00	18.63	56				
	02-04	04-XX	1	METHOTREXATE	30.00	19.95	56				
*				TOTALS	400.00	270.67	442	0.00	54.13	216.54	0.00

56 - Medicare limits payment to this amount.
442 - Total for these charges.

DETACH CHECK BEFORE CASHING

MEDICARE
1873 MONTROSE AVE
MINX, CO 82377

BANK OF COLORS (970) 555-5555
2300 Matchbox Way
Minx, CO 82377

04-9999
99-123
87654

February 27, 20 XX

PAY Three Thousand Four Hundred Sixteen and 44/100****************************** DOLLARS $ 3,416.44

TO
THE
ORDER
OF

Consolidated Health Services
1357 Castle Blvd, Suite 515
Colter, CO 81222-2222

Mike Medicarier

⑆0001111⑆ ⑈111000123⑈ 0123 4567⑆ ⑆00000011123⑆

ROVER INSURERS, INC.
5931 ROLLING ROAD
RONSON, CO 81369

PATIENT NAME	DATE OF SERVICE	PROCEDURE	BILLED AMOUNT	ALLOWED AMOUNT	% OF AMOUNT	PAYMENT AMOUNT	DENIED AMOUNT	REASON CODE
THEROAD, KENT C.	02/09/XX	ER VISIT	$ 150.00	$ 145.00	100%*	$ 125.00	$ 5.00	36
	02/09/XX	X-RAY ULNA	$ 30.00	$ 23.00	100%*	$ 23.00	$ 7.00	36
	TOTAL		$ 180.00	$ 168.00		$ 168.00	$ 12.00	
FORE-THEROAD, JUANA	02/09/XX	ER VISIT	$ 240.00	$ 215.00	100%*	$ 215.00	$ 25.00	36
	02/09/XX	X-RAY FAC	$ 50.00	$ 42.00	100%*	$ 42.00	$ 8.00	36
	02/09/XX	X-RAY SKULL	$ 85.00	$ 71.00	100%*	$ 71.00	$ 14.00	36
	02/09/XX	X-RAY SPINE	$ 40.00	$ 29.50	100%*	$ 29.50	$ 10.50	36
	02/09/XX	EMS DIRECT	$ 75.00	$ 60.00	100%*	$ 60.00	$ 15.00	36
	TOTAL		$ 490.00	$ 417.50		$ 417.50	$ 72.50	
THEROAD, IAN N.	02/09/XX	CRIT CARE	$ 600.00	$ 523.00	100%***	$ 500.00***	$ 77.00	36
	02/09/XX	MRI R THIGH	$ 700.00	$ 667.00	80%***	$ 432.00***	$ 33.00	36
	02/09/XX	X-RAY SKULL	$ 85.00	$ 71.00	80%	$ 56.80	$ 14.00	36
	02/09/XX	X-RAY SPINE	$ 100.00	$ 86.00	80%	$ 68.80	$ 14.00	36
	02/09/XX	X-RAY L LEG	$ 260.00	$ 209.00	80%	$ 167.20	$ 51.00	36
	02/09/XX	X-RAY R/L ARMS	$ 260.00	$ 219.00	80%	$ 175.20	$ 41.00	36
	02/09/XX	EMS DIRECT	$ 75.00	$ 60.00	80%	$ 48.00	$ 15.00	
	TOTAL		$2080.00	$1835.00		$1448.00	$245.00	
THEROAD, DONETTE	02/09/XX	ER VISIT	$ 45.00	$ 38.00	100%*	$ 38.00	$ 7.00	36
	TOTAL		$ 45.00	$ 38.00		$ 38.00	$ 7.00	
TOTALS			$2795.00	$2458.50		$2071.50	$336.50	

REASON CODES:
36   BILLED AMOUNT EXCEEDS AMOUNT ALLOWED BY THE PLAN.
*   ACCIDENT BENEFIT PAYS AT 100%
***   ACCIDENT BENEFIT APPLIES TO FIRST $500, DEDUCTIBLE TAKEN THEREAFTER.

DETACH CHECK BEFORE CASHING

ROVER INSURERS, INC.
5931 ROLLING ROAD
RONSON, CO 81369

BANK OF COLORS   (970) 555-5555
Ronson Branch
2300 Rocky Road
Ronson, CO 81369

04-10491

08-12
1100

March 17,   20 XX $ 2,071.50

PAY Two Thousand Seventy One and 50/100*** DOLLARS

TO
THE
ORDER
OF
Consolidated Health Services
1357 Castle Blvd, Suite 515
Colter, CO 81222-2222

Randy Rover
||0000011123||0

||001111||0 |:111000123|:   0123   4567||0

Document **44**

Billing Office,

Evan Lee Harps of 824 Pearly Way, Gates, CO, 82315, was declared brain dead at 8:05 am on 3/19/XX. He was involved in a motorcycle/auto accident, as the driver of the motorcycle. He was not wearing a helmet and received massive head injuries. His birthdate was 7/24/72. His Social Security number was 561-99-9615.

Please bill the insurances for Phillip D. Cupp for the following services performed by me, Butch M.N. Hackim, M.D.: Removal of Kidney for transplantation ($1,785) on 3/19/XX. The bill for the services to transplant the kidney into Phillip D. Cupp will be forthcoming at a later date, when follow-up care has been completed.

Dr. Anne S. Thesia, M.D. Anesthesiologist, has also asked that you bill Phillip D. Cupp's insurances for the administration of anesthesia during the above operation ($1,985). Anesthesia time: 3 hours 45 minutes.

Mr. Harps' wife authorized the release of information on 3/19/XX, as well as the assignment of benefits.

Thank you,

Butch M.N. Hackim, M.D.

Butch M.N. Hackim, M.D.

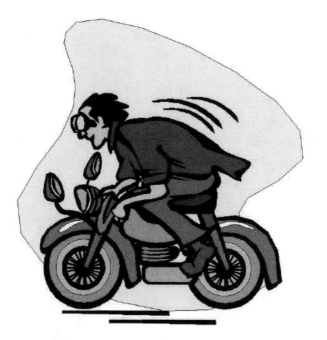

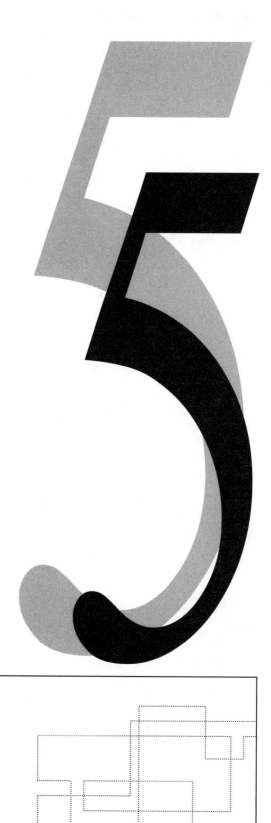

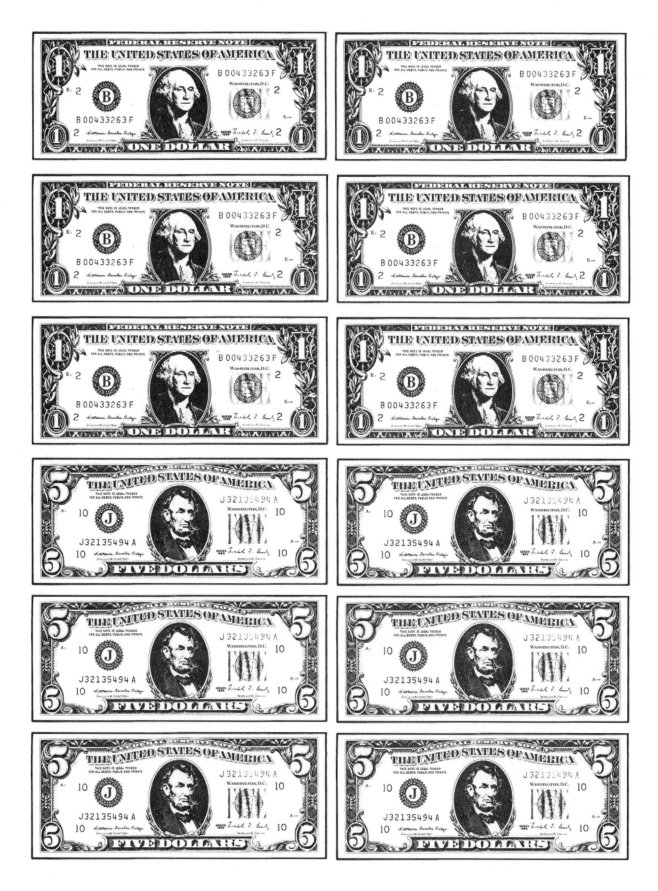

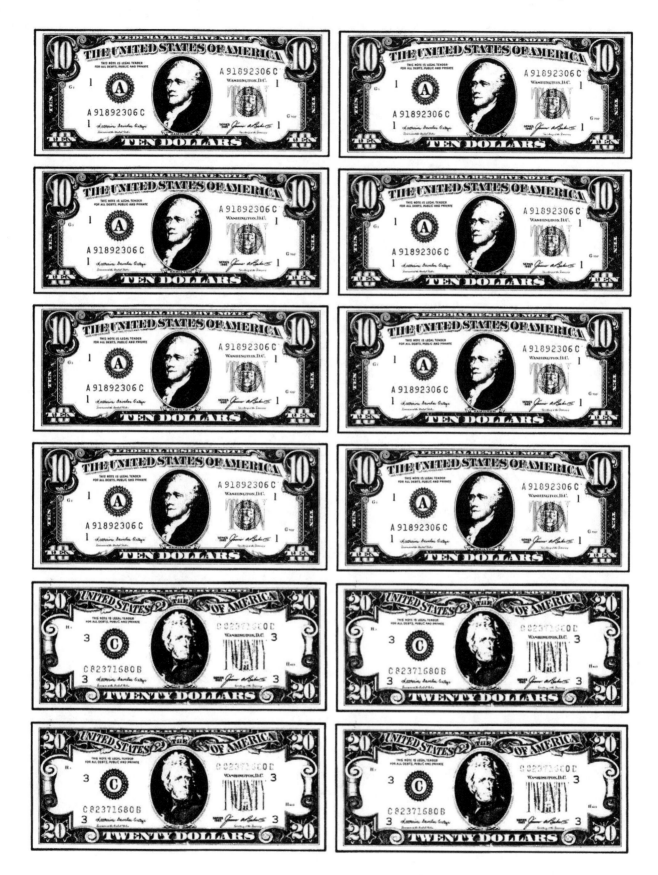

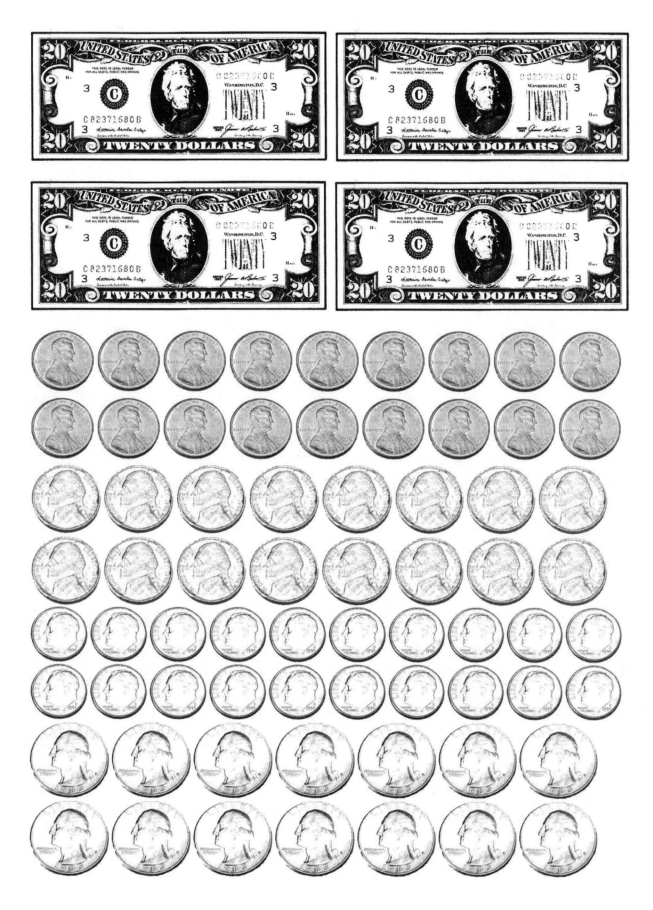

WINDOW PAYMENTS: The following payments were received at the billing office window or given with the claim information.

CLAIM 2 – Petey Attricks

SHERRY ATTRICKS   1932
RT 1 BOX 83   22-31
COLTER, CO 81235   1110

January 14   20 *XX*

Pay to the
order of   *Consolidated Health Services* $

_____ Dollars

SECOND BEST BANK
2223 SAHARA STREET
COLTER, CO 81221

For *Petey's visit*   *Sherry Attricks*

⑆11100011⑆ 230 0000 123456⑈

CLAIM 8 – Ima Knose   ### CLAIM 9 – Ron E. Knose

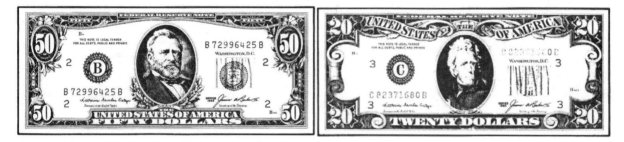

CLAIM 11 – Dee Pendent

ANDY PENDENT   2135
1111 E Dunphy Ave   11-00
Colter, CO 81222   1110

January 7   20 *XX*

Pay to the
order of *Consolidated Health Services* $ *350.00*

Three Hundred Fifty and 00/100------------------------------------- Dollars

THE BEST BANK
9012 BAKER BLVD.
COLTER, CO 81234

For *Dee Pendent's Hosp Stay*   *Andy Pendent*

⑆11100011⑆ 230 0000 123456⑈

CLAIM 14 – Barry Tired

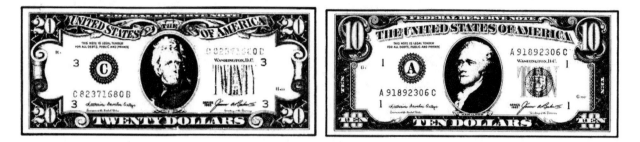

CLAIM 15 – V. Iris

D. JOBB DUNNITT   1805
160 ABERNATHY AVE #A   22-31
ARMSTRONG, CO 81569   1110

                                    January 19   20 *XX*

Pay to the
order of *Consolidated Health Services* | $

_____ Dollars

SECOND BEST BANK
2223 SAHARA STREET
COLTER, CO 81222

For *V. Iris's 1/21/XX Dr. Visit*   *D. Jobb Dunnitt*

|:11100011|: 230 0000 123456||▪

CLAIM 19 – Shay Kee Hart

SHAY KEE & BROOKE N. HART   1796
2093 GARDEN WAY   33-13
COLTER, CO 81223   1110

                                January 21   20 *XX*

Pay to the
order of *Consolidated Health Services* | $_____

_____ Dollars

THE BEST BANK
9012 BAKER BLVD.
COLTER, CO 81234

For *Medicare Ded & est pmt*   *Shay Kee Hart*

|:11100011|: 230 0000 123456||▪

CLAIM 26 – Sherry Attricks

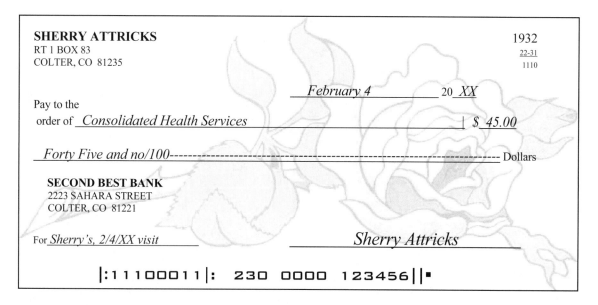

SHERRY ATTRICKS
RT 1 BOX 83
COLTER, CO 81235

1932

22-31
1110

February 4   20 XX

Pay to the
order of *Consolidated Health Services* $ 45.00

Forty Five and no/100--- Dollars

SECOND BEST BANK
2223 SAHARA STREET
COLTER, CO 81221

For *Sherry's, 2/4/XX visit*   *Sherry Attricks*

⑆11100011⑆ 230 0000 123456⑈

CLAIM 30 – Andy Pendent

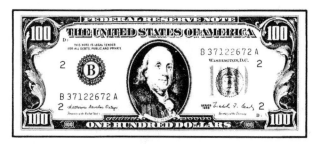

CLAIM 32 – D. Jobb Dunnitt

D. JOBB DUNNITT
160 ABERNATHY AVE #A
ARMSTRONG, CO 81569

1809

22-31
1110

January 23   20 XX

Pay to the
order of *Consolidated Health Services* $ 60.00

Sixty and 00/100-- Dollars

SECOND BEST BANK
2223 SAHARA STREET
COLTER, CO 81222

For *1/23/XX Hospital Visit*   *D. Jobb Dunnitt*

⑆11100011⑆ 230 0000 123456⑈

CLAIM 35 – Hugh Waite

HUGH WAITE   1298
222 BARKER BLVD.   33-13
COLTER, CO 81222   1110

                              January 11   20 *XX*

Pay to the
order of *Consolidated Health Services* | $ *400.00*

 Four Hundred and 00/100 -- Dollars

THIRD BEST BANK
3033 THIRD STREET
COLTER, CO 81333

For *Dr. Visit*   *Hugh Waite*

⑈11100011⑈: 230 0000 123456⑈

CLAIM 36 – Shay Kee Hart

SHAY KEE & BROOKE N. HART   1835
2093 GARDEN WAY   33-13
COLTER, CO 81223   1110

                              February 2   20 *XX*

Pay to the
order of *Consolidated Health Services* | $_____

_____ Dollars

THE BEST BANK
9012 BAKER BLVD.
COLTER, CO 81234

For *Est payment dr visit 2/4/XX*   *Shay Kee Hart*

⑈11100011⑈: 230 0000 123456⑈

CLAIM 37 – Cass N. O'Gen

PAT N. O'GEN   2938
621 CAYHILL AVE.   22-31
COLTER, CO 81222   1110

                              January 29   20 *XX*

Pay to the
order of *Consolidated Health Services* | $ *125.00*

 One Hundred Twenty Five and no/100-- Dollars

SECOND BEST BANK
2223 SAHARA STREET
COLTER, CO 81221

For *Dr. visit*   *Pat N. O'Gen*

⑈11100011⑈: 230 0000 123456⑈

CLAIM 39 – Ron E. Knose

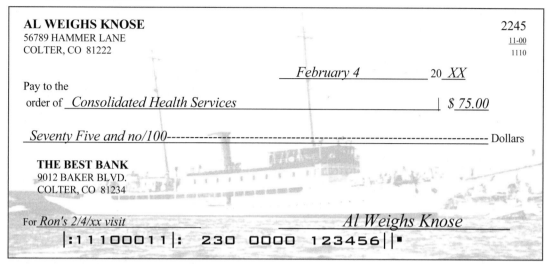

AL WEIGHS KNOSE
56789 HAMMER LANE
COLTER, CO 81222

2245

11-00
1110

February 4   20 *XX*

Pay to the
order of *Consolidated Health Services* | $ *75.00*

Seventy Five and no/100-- Dollars

THE BEST BANK
9012 BAKER BLVD.
COLTER, CO 81234

For *Ron's 2/4/xx visit*   *Al Weighs Knose*

|:11100011|: 230 0000 123456||•

CLAIM 52 – Jeanette Akenja-Nearing

**Jeanette Akenja-Nearing
& Gene Poole**
4738 JESSUP ROAD
JASPER, CO 81335

1815

33-13
1110

February 29   20 *XX*

Pay to the
order of *Consolidated Health Services* | $ *1,500.00*

One Thousand Five Hundred Dollars and 00/100----------------------------------- Dollars

THIRD BEST BANK
3033 THIRD STREET
COLTER, CO 81333

For *Maternity Care*   *Jeanette Akenja-Nearing*

|:11100011|: 230 0000 123456||•

CLAIM 60 – Beane Andy Knose

AL WEIGHS KNOSE
56789 HAMMER LANE
COLTER, CO 81222

2261

11-00
1110

March 2   20 *XX*

Pay to the
order of *Consolidated Health Services* | $ *50.00*

Fifty and 00/100-- Dollars

THE BEST BANK
9012 BAKER BLVD.
COLTER, CO 81234

For *Pmt in full for all medical svcs*   *Al Weighs Knose*

|:11100011|: 230 0000 123456||•

CLAIM 102 – Jose Fraide

B. A. and Nada Fraide
9009 Marble Manor Lane
COLTON, CO 81956

3003
11-00
1110

January 15   20 XX

Pay to the
order of *Consolidated Health Services* | $ 15.00

Fifteen and 00/100-- Dollars

THE BEST BANK
9012 BAKER BLVD.
COLTER, CO 81234

For *Office visit*   *Nada Fraide*

|:1 1 1 0 0 0 1 1|:   2 3 0   0 0 0 0   1 2 3 4 5 6||▪

CLAIM 103 – Jose Fraide

B. A. and Nada Fraide
9009 Marble Manor Lane
COLTON, CO 81956

3004
11-00
1110

January 15   20 XX

Pay to the
order of *Consolidated Health Services* | $ 15.00

Fifteen and 00/100-- Dollars

THE BEST BANK
9012 BAKER BLVD.
COLTER, CO 81234

For *Office visit*   *Nada Fraide*

|:1 1 1 0 0 0 1 1|:   2 3 0   0 0 0 0   1 2 3 4 5 6||▪

CLAIM 104 – Jose Fraide

B. A. and Nada Fraide
9009 Marble Manor Lane
COLTON, CO 81956

3016
11-00
1110

February 25   20 XX

Pay to the
order of *Consolidated Health Services* | $ 15.00

Fifteen and 00/100-- Dollars

THE BEST BANK
9012 BAKER BLVD.
COLTER, CO 81234

For *Office visit*   *Nada Fraide*

|:1 1 1 0 0 0 1 1|:   2 3 0   0 0 0 0   1 2 3 4 5 6||▪

Patient File Forms

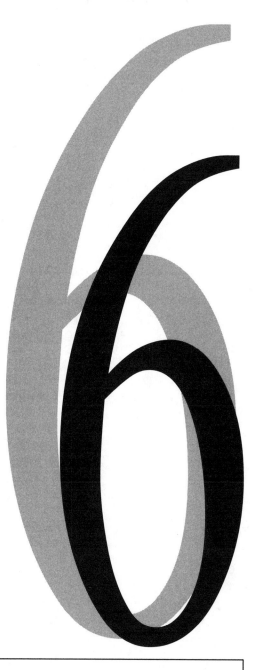

Following are the file forms you will need if you are completing some or all of the Simulated Work Program in a manual format. One copy of each of the forms has been provided here. While these forms are copyrighted by ICDC Publishing, Inc., purchase of this text allows you the right to copy these forms as needed to complete the Simulated Work Program assignments.

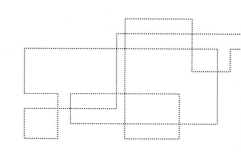

PATIENT INFORMATION SHEET

INSURED'S INFORMATION

Patient ID: _____ Assigned Provider: _____ Birth date: _____

Name: (Last, First, Middle) _____ Sex: _____

Address: (Inc City, State, Zip) _____

Home Phone: _____ Marital Status:_____ Social Security #: _____

Employer Name: _____ Work Phone: _____

Employer Address: _____

Employment Status: _____ Referred by: _____

Allergies/Medical conditions: _____

Primary Ins Name: _____ Address: _____

ID #: _____ Plan #/Name: _____ Policy Holder Name: _____

Secondary Ins Name: _____ Address: _____

ID #: _____ Plan #/Name: _____ Policy Holder Name: _____

SPOUSE'S INFORMATION

Patient ID: _____ Assigned Provider: _____ Birth date: _____

Name: (Last, First, Middle) _____ Sex: _____

Social Security #: _____ Employment Status:_____

Employer Name: _____ Work Phone: _____

Employer Address: _____

Allergies/Medical conditions: _____

Primary Ins Name: _____ Address: _____

ID #: _____ Plan #/Name: _____ Policy Holder Name: _____

Secondary Ins Name: _____ Address: _____

ID #: _____ Plan #/Name: _____ Policy Holder Name: _____

CHILD #1

Patient ID: _____ Assigned Provider: _____ Birth date: _____

Name of Minor Child: _____ Social Security #: _____

Sex: _____ Marital Status: _____ Relationship to Insured: _____

Allergies/Medical conditions: _____

Primary Ins Name: _____ Primary Insured: _____

Secondary Ins Name: _____ Secondary Insured: _____

CHILD #2

Patient ID: _____ Assigned Provider: _____ Birth date: _____

Name of Minor Child: _____ Social Security #: _____

Sex: _____ Marital Status: _____ Relationship to Insured: _____

Allergies/Medical conditions: _____

Primary Ins Name: _____ Primary Insured: _____

Secondary Ins Name: _____ Secondary Insured: _____

EMERGENCY CONTACT

Name: _____ Home Phone: _____ Other Phone: _____

Address: (Inc City, State, Zip)_____

ACKNOWLEDGMENT AND AUTHORITY FOR TREATMENT AND PAYMENT

Initial

_____ I consent to treatment as necessary or desirable to the care of the patient named above, including but not restricted to whatever drugs, medicine, performance of operations and conduct of laboratory, x-ray, or other studies that may be used by the attending doctor, his/her nurse or qualified designate:

_____ I also acknowledge full responsibility for the payment of such services and agree to pay for them upon demand, in full, AT THE TIME OF SERVICE. If the physician must use a collection agency/attorney or court to collect its charges, then I will pay reasonable attorney fees and costs incurred in collecting same, regardless of insurance coverage.

_____ I hereby authorize payment directly to Consolidated Health Services of the medical expense benefits otherwise payable to me but not to exceed my indebtedness to said physician on account of the enclosed charge.

_____ I hereby authorize any medical practitioner, medical or medically related facility, insurance or reinsuring company, consumer reporting agency, or employer having information with respect to any physical or mental condition and/or treatment of me or my minor children and any other non-medical information of me and my minor children to give to the group policy holder, my employer, or its legal representative, any and all such information.

_____ I understand the information obtained by the use of the Authorization will be used to determine eligibility for insurance, and eligibility for benefits under any existing policy. Any information obtained will not be released by/to any organization EXCEPT to the group policyholder, my employer, reinsuring companies, the Medical Information Bureau, Inc., or other persons or organizations performing business or legal services in connection with my application, claim, or as may be otherwise lawfully required or as I may further authorize.

_____ I further agree that a photographic copy of this Authorization shall be valid as the original. This Authorization shall be valid for one year from the date shown below.

Signature of Insured: _____ Date: _____

Signature of Spouse: _____ Date: _____

RECEIPT

Date _____ 19 _____ No. _____

Received From _____

Address _____

_____ Dollars $ _____

For _____

ACCOUNT			HOW PAID		
AMT. OF ACCOUNT			CASH		
AMT. PAID			CHECK		
BALANCE DUE			MONEY ORDER		

By _____

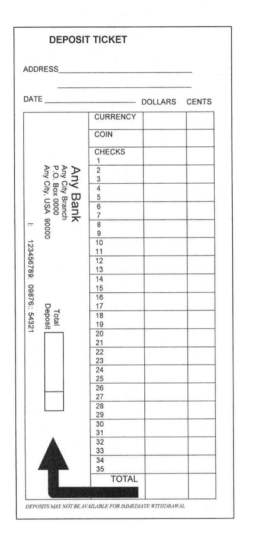

DEPOSIT TICKET

ADDRESS _____

_____

DATE _____ DOLLARS CENTS

Any Bank
Any City Branch
P.O. Box 0000
Any City, USA 90000

⑆ 123456789⑆ 09876⑈ 54321

	DOLLARS	CENTS
CURRENCY		
COIN		
CHECKS		
1		
2		
3		
4		
5		
6		
7		
8		
9		
10		
11		
12		
13		
14		
15		
16		
17		
18		
19		
20		
21		
22		
23		
24		
25		
26		
27		
28		
29		
30		
31		
32		
33		
34		
35		
TOTAL		

Total Deposit

DEPOSITS MAY NOT BE AVAILABLE FOR IMMEDIATE WITHDRAWAL

PETTY CASH COUNT

DATE _____

TIME _____

	QUANTITY	AMOUNT
CURRENCY		
$100	_____	_____
$50	_____	_____
$20	_____	_____
$10	_____	_____
$5	_____	_____
$1	_____	_____
TOTAL		_____
COINS		
$1	_____	_____
Half $	_____	_____
Quarters	_____	_____
Dimes	_____	_____
Nickels	_____	_____
Pennies	_____	_____
TOTAL		_____
RECEIPTS TOTAL +		_____
GRAND TOTAL		_____

PETTY CASH RECEIPT

RECEIVED OF PETTY CASH

NUMBER _____ DATE _____

AMOUNT _____

FOR _____

_____

_____

CHARGE TO ACCOUNT _____

_____ _____
APPROVED BY   RECEIVED BY

Ledger Card

RESPONSIBLE PARTY: _____

ADDRESS: _____

TELEPHONE #: _____

PATIENT NAME: _____ PATIENT #: _____

SPECIAL NOTES: _____

Date	Description of Service	Charge	Payments	Adjustments	Remaining Balance

Daily Journal

Date	Name	Description of Services	Charge	Payments	Adjustments	Remaining Balance

CONSOLIDATED HEALTH SERVICES

Medical Billing Office
1357 Castle Blvd., Suite 515
Colter, CO 81222
(970) 555-4567

Serving all your medical needs for 17 years

CONSOLIDATED HEALTH SERVICES

Medical Billing Office
1357 Castle Blvd., Suite 515
Colter, CO 81222
(970) 555-4567

Date: _____

Re: Policy Holder: _____

Control: _____

Employee: _____

Dependent: _____

Dear _____ :

We need additional information from you.

We are writing to _____

_____

_____

_____

_____

_____

Please respond on the reverse of this letter or attach additional information or documentation. Thank you.

Sincerely yours,

Policyholder copy enclosed

Serving all your medical needs for 17 years!

Charge Slip

Date of Service: _____   Account Number: _____

Name (Last, First): _____

X	Code	Description	Fee	X	Code	Description	Fee	X	Code	Description	Fee
Initial				**Established**				**Special Procedures**			
	99204	Extended Exam	100.00		99211	Minimal Exam	35.00				
	99205	Comprehensive Exam	110.00		99212	Brief Exam	40.00				
					99213	Limited Exam	45.00				
					99214	Intermediate Exam	60.00				
					99215	Comprehensive Exam	90.00				
Consultations				**Laboratory**				**Prescriptions**			
	99244	Comprehensive	150.00		36415	Venipuncture	15.00				
					81000	Urinalysis	10.00				
					82948	Glucose Fingerstick	18.00				

X	Code	Diagnosis	X	Code	Diagnosis	X	Code	Diagnosis
	466	Bronchitis, Acute		401	Hypertension		460	Upper Resp Tract Infection
	428	Congestive Heart Failure		414	Ischemic Heart Disease		599.0	Urinary Tract Infection
	431	CVA		724.2	Low Back Syndrome		616	Vaginitis
	250.0	Diabetes Mellitus		278.0	Obesity		**ICD-9**	**Other Diagnosis**
	625.3	Dysmenorrhea		715	Osteoarthritis			
	345	Epilepsy		462	Pharyngitis. Acute			
	0009.0	Gastroenteritis		714	Rheumatoid Arthritis			
	784.0	Headache		477	Rhinitis, Allergic			
	573.3	Hepatitis		471	Sinusitis. Acute			

Remarks/Special Instructions	New Appointment	Statement of Account	
		Old Balance	
		Today's Fee	
Referring Physician	Recall	Payment	
		New Balance	

Insurance Claims Register

Page No. _____

Date Claims Filed	Patient Name	Name of Insurance	Place Claim Sent	Claim Amount	Follow-Up Date	Paid Amount	Remaining Balance

Authorized Treatment Form

Patient Name: _____

Policy Name: _____

Above patient has been authorized for the following treatment(s):

    Diagnosis: _____

    Authorized Procedure(s): _____

    Allowed Number of Treatments: _____

    Treatment Authorized by: _____

    Treatment Authorization Number: _____

TREATMENT RECORD

Visit	Date	Procedure(s)	Provider
1	_____	_____	_____
2	_____	_____	_____
3	_____	_____	_____
4	_____	_____	_____
5	_____	_____	_____
6	_____	_____	_____
7	_____	_____	_____
8	_____	_____	_____
9	_____	_____	_____
10	_____	_____	_____
11	_____	_____	_____
12	_____	_____	_____
13	_____	_____	_____
14	_____	_____	_____
15	_____	_____	_____
16	_____	_____	_____
17	_____	_____	_____
18	_____	_____	_____
19	_____	_____	_____
20	_____	_____	_____

Patient Aging

Patient	Current	31 – 60 Days	61 – 90 Days	91+ Days	Total

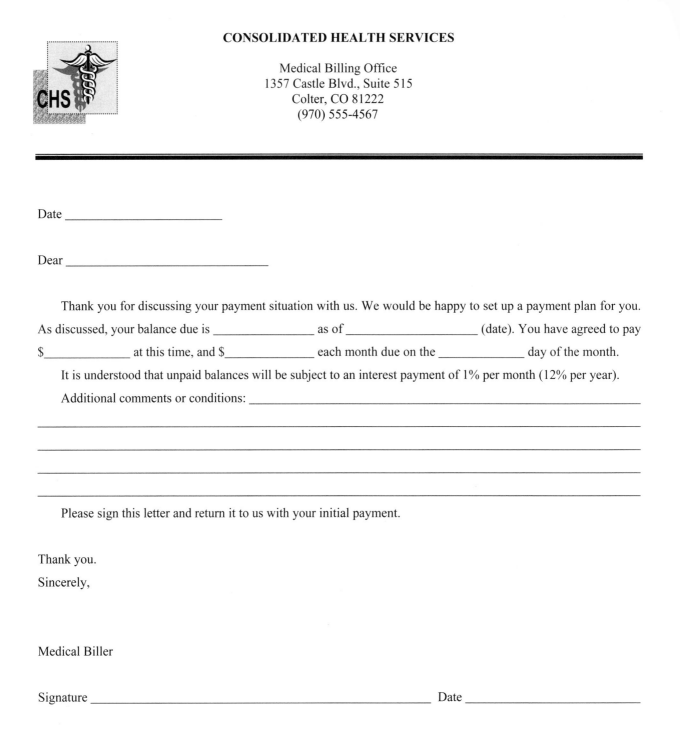

CONSOLIDATED HEALTH SERVICES

Medical Billing Office
1357 Castle Blvd., Suite 515
Colter, CO 81222
(970) 555-4567

Date _____

Dear _____

     Thank you for discussing your payment situation with us. We would be happy to set up a payment plan for you. As discussed, your balance due is _____ as of _____ (date). You have agreed to pay $_____ at this time, and $_____ each month due on the _____ day of the month.

     It is understood that unpaid balances will be subject to an interest payment of 1% per month (12% per year).

     Additional comments or conditions: _____

_____

_____

_____

_____

     Please sign this letter and return it to us with your initial payment.

Thank you.

Sincerely,

Medical Biller

Signature _____ Date _____

Serving all your medical needs for 17 years!

Insurance Coverage Sheet

INSURED: _____ BIRTHDATE: _____

SSN: _____ EFFECTIVE DATE: _____

DEDUCTIBE AMOUNT: _____ 3 MO CARRYOVER?: _____ COINSURANCE%: _____

FAMILY DEDUCTIBLE: _____ AGGREGATE/NON-AGGREGATE

DEPENDENT AGE LIMIT: _____

BENEFITS PAID AT OTHER THAN THE STANDARD COINSURANCE % [Including benefit, coinsurance amount and special circumstances, (i.e., SSO allowed at 100%, required for hysterectomy, coronary bypass, etc.)]:

_____

_____

_____

_____

_____

PRE-AUTHORIZATION REQUIRED FOR: _____

_____

_____

ACCIDENT BENEFIT AMOUNT: _____ TREATMENT TO BE RECEIVED WITHIN _____ DAYS

OTHER NOTES/COMMENTS: _____

_____

_____

_____

_____

Total Payments (20XX)

Indicate below the names of the insured and their dependents. When any of the following information is received, write it in pencil followed by the date. This will help you to realize when a patient's deductible has been met and if they are nearing any maximum benefits.

	INSURED	DEPENDENT	DEPENDENT	DEPENDENT	DEPENDENT
NAME:	_____	_____	_____	_____	_____
DEDUCTIBE:	_____	_____	_____	_____	_____
COINS PD:	_____	_____	_____	_____	_____
LIFETIME:	_____	_____	_____	_____	_____

GUIDE TO MEDICAL BILLING

ICDC Publishing's Guide to Medical Billing textbook, along with its companion workbook provides a thorough understanding of the job skills covered. We specialize in easy-to-understand texts that cover every topic or skill needed to learn to competently handle the job. Filled with practical advice and hands-on activities, this text provides a complete understanding of all the skills needed to perform as a medical biller.

ICDC Publishing specializes in textbooks and workbooks with a difference!

Table of Contents:

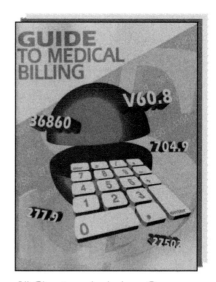

All Chapters include a Summary of Key Points, a List of Assignments, Questions for Review, Exercises, and an Honors Certification™.

Trade Paperback, pp. 335:
ISBN: 1-881159-14-0

To order this book, or for a list of all our titles, and to see complete **Tables of Contents** and **Sample Chapters**, visit our website at:

www.icdcpublishing.com